Food, bacteria and health
A practical guide

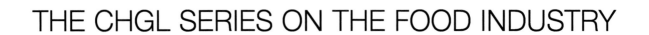

THE CHGL SERIES ON THE FOOD INDUSTRY

Food, bacteria and health
A practical guide

Carol Phillips

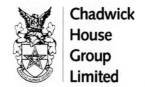
Chadwick
House
Group
Limited

ISBN 1-902423-49-6

© Carol Phillips

Chadwick House Group Limited
Chadwick Court
15 Hatfields
London
SE1 8DG
England

Publications Tel: 020 7827 5882
Fax: 020 7827 9930
Email: Publications@chgl.com
www.cieh.org

Chadwick House Group Ltd is the trading subsidiary of the Chartered Institute of Environmental Health (CIEH), the professional and educational body for those who work in environmental health in England, Wales and Northern Ireland. Founded in 1883, the Chartered Institute has charitable status and its primary function is the promotion of knowledge and understanding of environmental health issues.

Dedication

To my husband and daughter, without whose encouragement and patience this book would not have been written.

Contents

Acknowledgements

I would like to thank all those who helped prepare the manuscript of this book, especially colleagues in the IT department at Nene-University College, Northampton who painstakingly helped me with the use of word processing packages and taught me the value of saving copies of documents on more than one computer disk. Particular thanks go to Ms Susan Maloney for her help with the final preparation of the camera ready copy.

The Author

The author completed her BSc and PhD in Microbiology at Cardiff University. After some years in the pathology department of a busy hospital she entered academic life. She is now a lecturer at Nene-University College, Northampton where she has an active research programme in food microbiology, with emphasis on *Campylobacter* and related organisms.
(E.MAIL. CAROL.PHILLIPS@NENE.AC.UK)

CHAPTER 1

BACTERIAL FOOD-POISONING AS A PUBLIC HEALTH ISSUE

1.1. Introduction

Food and its safety have become a major concern of both governments and consumers in recent years. The effect of loss of confidence in the safety of food has major consequences for the food industry and the individual. The *'E. coli* O157 in beef' scare that received a great deal of media attention in late 1996 and early 1997 clearly showed this to be the case.

The numbers of food-poisoning incidents reported by The Public Health Laboratory Service (PHLS) Communicable Disease Surveillance Centre (CDSC) (in excess of 90 000 in 1997) have a massive resource implication within the NHS and the community as a whole. Each case of food poisoning caused by the bacterium *Campylobacter*, for example, has been estimated to cost the country more than £500 if the intangible costs of pain and suffering are included and there were 50 247 such cases in 1997. The investigation of the means by which such organisms spread into, and within, the food chain is an important aspect of improving food safety.

This introductory chapter defines food-poisoning and examines various aspects of an increasing major public health problem. It includes sections on how the statistics are compiled and what they mean, the trends over the last decade, the main causes of food-borne illness and the symptoms they cause together with a brief description of the Hazard Analysis and Critical Control Point (HACCP) concept. The book as a whole attempts to give a broad outline of the bacterial pathogens found in food and their effects on human health. It also explores some ways in which food safety issues are addressed by food producers and legislators.

1.2. Definition of food-poisoning

In 1992 the Chief Medical Officer for England and Wales circulated all doctors with the following definition of food-poisoning which had already been adopted by the World Health Organisation: **food-poisoning is any disease of an infectious or toxic nature caused by or thought to be caused by the consumption of food or water**.

This definition encompasses **all** food-borne and water-borne illnesses including those that cause symptoms other than those related to the gastrointestinal tract. Illnesses caused by toxic chemicals are **included** but illnesses which may produce gastrointestinal symptoms but are caused by an immunological response such as food allergies are **excluded**.

There are many different types of food poisoning caused by both micro-organisms and by other contamination of food (Table 1.1.). Many foods contain substances which can be toxic to humans when consumed in large quantities. Some vitamins, for example, although beneficial in the correct quantities, may prove toxic if consumed in excess. Other foods may contain toxins due to the conversion of naturally occurring compound in the food. One example is the alkaloid, solanine, found in green potatoes after inappropriate storage conditions.

Table 1.1. Possible causes of food poisoning.

Microbial infection / intoxication

bacterial e.g. *Campylobacter / Staphylococcus*

protozoal e.g. *Cryptosporidium*

viral e.g. small round structured virus (SRSV)

fungal e.g. aflavotoxins formed by *Aspergillus*

Microbial spoilage

scombroid poisoning from bacterial spoilage of fish

Poisonous animals

ciguatera poisoning from tropical and sub-tropical fish following their consumption of poisonous dinoflagellates

Poisonous plants

deadly nightshade

Chemicals

heavy metals e.g. copper, mercury, thallium

pesticides e.g. chlordane

preservatives (in excess) e.g. nitrates, nitrites

1.3. Bacterial causes of food-poisoning or food-borne illness

The problems in collating data on gastrointestinal disease overall are many and various. Further determining whether the illness was food-borne or not additionally complicates the statistical analysis concerning the numbers and types of food poisoning which occur in any country. In terms of numbers, microbiological agents, particularly bacteria (Table 1.2.), are the major cause of reported gastrointestinal illness. In the majority of countries the most detailed information is collated on bacterial food-associated pathogens.

Table 1.2. Major bacterial causes of food-associated illness.

Bacterium	Food vehicle identified
Aeromonas	mainly water-borne
Arcobacter	pork
Bacillus cereus	cooked rice, cooked meats
Campylobacter species	poultry, raw milk
Clostridium botulinum	fish, meat, canned vegetables
Clostridium perfringens	gravy, cooked meat, poultry
Escherichia coli	
Enterotoxigenic (ETEC)	raw vegetables, salads
Enteropathogenic (EPEC)	milk
Enteroinvasive (EIEC)	cheese
Enterhaemorrhagic (EHEC)	undercooked meat, particularly beef,
Listeria monocytogenes	soft cheeses, coleslaw, pate
Salmonella typhi	vegetable salads, meat and meat products, dairy products
Salmonella (non-*typhi*)	meat, milk, eggs, dairy products
Shigella	potato/egg salads
Staphylococcus aureus	ham, poultry, eggs, dairy products, ice-cream
Vibrio species	shellfish
Yersinia enterocolitica	milk, poultry, pork, fish

1.4. Compilation of food-poisoning statistics in England and Wales

Surveillance of food-borne illness in England and Wales is the responsibility of the Communicable Disease Surveillance Centre (CDSC).

4

The objectives of surveillance are:

- early detection of outbreaks so that they may be promptly investigated and controlled
- monitoring long term trends to assess the need for intervention
- evaluating the effectiveness of control measures
- identification of prevalent infectious agents and dissemination of such information to clinicians to help in the accurate and immediate diagnosis of cause of illness and hence treatment
- national collation of data on rare or emerging causes of food-borne illness to enable research to be carried out on such causes.

There are five main elements involved in surveillance

- systematic collection of data from all available sources
- analysis of data obtained to produce statistics
- interpretation of data in terms of identifying trends
- distribution of statistics and interpretation to public health workers who are enabled to act in an appropriate way
- evaluation of preventative measures.

CDSC receives information routinely on laboratory confirmed infections and general outbreaks of infectious intestinal disease from national surveillance schemes. The collection of data from these sources allows the CDSC to monitor closely trends in gastrointestinal disease overall and particularly cases caused by bacterial pathogens.

The following terms are used in reporting the statistics and data on food-poisoning in England and Wales (and in Scotland and Northern Ireland):

- a **case** is a person with symptoms from whom a recognised pathogen has been isolated
- an **outbreak** is two or more cases which may be either **family** or **general**

- a **sporadic case** is a person with symptoms but with no known association with another case
- an **incident** is either a sporadic case or an outbreak
- a **notification** is a case reported by a doctor and clinically confirmed
- **otherwise ascertained cases** are those suspected but not notified.

Otherwise ascertained cases may occur for various reasons. For example, a notification may be made by a microbiologist after laboratory isolation of a pathogen from a clinical specimen from a patient who has not been formally notified by a doctor as a food-poisoning case. Environmental Health Officers (EHOs) may also discover previously unrecognised cases while investigating an outbreak of gastrointestinal disease.

1.4.1. Notification of food poisoning

Statutes require all doctors in clinical practice to notify the proper officer of the local authority who is generally the consultant in communicable disease control (CCDC). If an illness is covered by the definition of food-poisoning but is also in itself a notifiable disease, such as typhoid, for example, then it is reported specifically as that disease and not as food-poisoning.

The *Public Health (Infectious Diseases) Regulations 1988* require notifications made by the physician attending the patient suspected of illness to include data such as name, age and gender of the suspected case to be sent to the 'proper officer' of the local authority, usually the Consultant in Communicable Disease Control of the relevant District Health Authority. Prompt notification is encouraged (to which is attached a fee) and should not depend on laboratory confirmation of the case. This results in a more efficient investigation of the source of infection and prevention of further spread of illness in the community.

Both formally notified and otherwise ascertained cases are collated and reported on a weekly basis. This data is published by CDSC in *Communicable Disease Report* and is also available on the CDSC world wide web home page. Local authorities are obliged to amend figures to CDSC on a quarterly and annual basis if there are any discrepancies due to further investigations of cases proving them to be not food-borne but because of person to person or animal to person spread.

The number of food-poisoning notifications (both formal and otherwise ascertained) has risen annually for the last decade, especially since 1992 (Figure 1.1.) which may be attributable to the general circulation to clinicians of the new definition. However, as in other countries, there is under-reporting of cases which may be caused by various factors:

- individuals with transient symptoms not reporting them to a clinician
- clinicians not being aware of legal requirement for notification
- clinicians not being aware of the importance of notification.

It is generally accepted that notifications therefore only provide an approximation of the total burden of food-borne illness to the NHS and the community at large with some estimates suggesting that as few as 10% of all cases are notified (Figure 1.2.).

Figure 1.1. Annual corrected food-poisoning notifications (compiled from CDSC statistics).

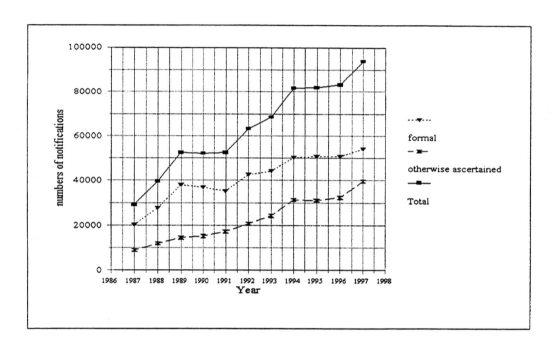

Figure 1.2. Notified cases represent only a proportion of actual cases of food-poisoning
(Wall et al, 1996: Reproduced with permission of PHLS CDSC).

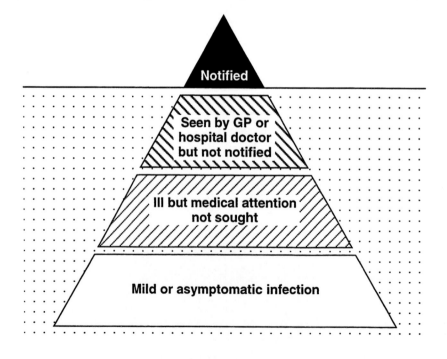

1.4.2. National surveillance scheme for laboratory confirmed infections

CDSC, the epidemiology unit of the PHLS, receives reports of laboratory confirmed cases of human infections from more than 250 laboratories throughout England and Wales including all local and reference laboratories and from NHS laboratories. The *Strategic Review of Pathology Services* in 1995 recommended that 'all pathology contracts should refer to the necessity for prompt reporting of data relevant to the epidemiology of communicable disease both to CCDC (i.e. local authority consultant of communicable disease control) and to the PHLS CDSC'.

CDSC generates, either by electronic reports from the outlying laboratories or, to a much lesser extent, via manual input, a database 'LabBase' which contains reports on approximately 400 species, subspecies and types of organisms including gastrointestinal pathogens such as *Salmonella* species. The Laboratory for Enteric Pathogens (LEP) also has an input into LabBase since **all** human isolates of *Salmonella* should be sent to it for confirmation and typing to genus level. The Salmonella figures are updated on a daily basis. Laboratories are encouraged as part of an extensive research programme on the sources and risk factors involved in other gastrointestinal infections such as *Escherichia coli* O157 and *Campylobacter* to send isolates of these organisms to LEP for further identification. LabBase can monitor changes in current trends thus allowing early detection of outbreaks.

Historical patterns are used to calculate exceedance scores which will indicate if the incidence of a particular organism is exceeding what would be expected for a particular week of the year. An exceedance score is calculated using the formula:

Exceedance score = observed total - expected total / threshold - expected total

The system works as an early warning since if this exceedance score is more than 1 then it suggests that there may be an outbreak of infection of that particular organism.

Gastrointestinal pathogens account for nearly 50% of all laboratory reports to CDSC but even this probably represents only a fraction of the true incidence. Only some of those individuals infected will experience transient symptoms and only a proportion of those will visit their general practitioner or another doctor. Not all of these will have specimens taken and some of these will test negative because of various factors such as the low level of infection or because of the time involved before they are examined. Even a positive result will not necessarily be reported to CDSC although the possibility of this occurring is reducing as the system becomes embedded (Figure 1.3.). A study in 1996, in a small number of GP practices, confirmed under-reporting was occurring to some extent. In the study it was found that only about one in 26 people who suffer an acute bout of gastrointestinal illness actually consults medical advice.

Figure 1.3. Laboratory reports collated by the CDSC only represent a proportion of actual cases (Wall et al, 1996: reproduced with permission PHLS CDSC).

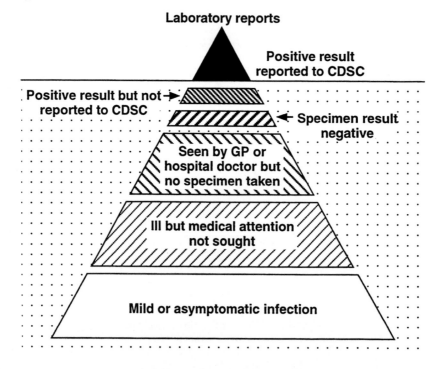

Changes in detection and reporting protocols and efficiencies in diagnostic procedures influence the incidence of certain pathogens as reported to CDSC. So-called 'emerging' pathogens such as *Escherichia coli* O157 may appear to increase in incidence but in fact the true nature of any increase is masked by an increased testing rate, in this case recommended by the Advisory Committee for Microbiological Safety of Food (ACMSF) in 1995. Since no data is available to CDSC on the number and type of negative samples tested in each laboratory, local and regional differences in testing efficiencies are not evident on LabBase making apparent differences in regional incidences difficult to interpret.

1.4.3. National surveillance scheme for general outbreaks of infectious intestinal disease

A general outbreak is defined as 'an outbreak which affects individuals from more than one private residence or which affects more than one individual from an institution'. Surveillance of general outbreaks has taken place since 1992 by CDSC who are informed of the possibility of such outbreaks from many sources including EHOs, general practitioners, clinical microbiologists and CCDCs. Investigations of general outbreaks involve collection of data concerning the pathogen involved, the source of the infection and the means of spread within the community. Usually evidence for the source of infection cannot be confirmed by laboratory testing because, for example, the suspected food vehicle has been consumed or otherwise disposed of, so evidence may be circumstantial or anecdotal. Data is used to formulate policies concerning control and prevention. However, although CDSC requests the investigating agent to complete a questionnaire concerning the outbreak, this is not a mandatory requirement. This results in some outbreaks not being identified, especially if they are spread over a wide area as often happens with a contaminated retail product.

Food-borne general outbreaks represent only a small number of the total laboratory reports

11

(Table 1.3.). The remainder may be family outbreaks, authentic sporadic cases or cases which are linked to general outbreaks which have not been recognised or reported as such.

Table 1.3. General outbreaks as a proportion of total laboratory reports in England and Wales, 1992-4 (compiled from CDSC statistics).

Organism	Percentage of laboratory confirmed cases occurring in general outbreaks
Salmonella spp.	6.0
Campylobacter spp.	0.2
Shigella sonnei	0.3
Clostridium perfringens	27.0
Escherichia coli O157	10.0

1.4.4. Conclusion

The CDSC collates information from the different sources, analyses data in terms of trends etc. and disseminates the results to those who are authorised to take appropriate action such as local health authorities or EHOs. The information from the different sources may be regarded as incomplete individually with each having advantages and disadvantages (Table 1.4.) but considered as a whole they probably provide a true reflection of the incidence of food-associated pathogens in England and Wales.

Table 1.4. Advantages and disadvantages of the sources from which statistics are compiled.

Source	Advantages	Disadvantages
Notifications	Does not depend on laboratory confirmation	Under-notification because doctors not aware of legal requirement/ importance of notification
National surveillance scheme for laboratory confirmed infections	Early detection of potential outbreaks; accurate typing of organisms	Only laboratory **confirmed** cases included; changes in testing requirements/sensitivity over time not taken into account
National surveillance scheme for general outbreaks of infectious intestinal disease	Provides data for development of preventative and control measures within the community	Widely dispersed outbreaks may not be recognised; classification (food-borne v. person to person) subjective; only represents a proportion of actual cases

1.5. Epidemiology of food-borne illness

Comparisons of statistics on food-poisoning cases between countries are difficult to assess because of the different reporting regimes and their relative efficiency. For example, in the

USA, because reporting of food-borne illness to the Center for Infectious Diseases is not compulsory, different states appear to have many times more cases than others. In the early 1980s, Canada, which has a much smaller population than the USA (approximately 10%), appeared, if official statistics were regarded as a true reflection of actual cases of food-poisoning, to have roughly five times as many cases per 100 000 population than theUSA. There might be two explanations for this discrepancy: either the Canadian population is much more susceptible to food-borne illness than that of the USA or, which is a more likely scenario, that there is a massive under-reporting in the USA. Also, during the 1970s and 1980s the CDC was able to determine the causative agent in only 45 to 55% of the food outbreaks examined.

In European countries too there is a similar problem concerning different national systems for notification and reporting of outbreaks which means that comparison of data from different countries is difficult and often meaningless. Different systems include:

- notification of cases of food-borne disease without specification of causative agent or any other epidemiological data
- reporting only **laboratory-confirmed** cases collated by a central agency
- reporting **all** cases of gastrointestinal disease whether or not they are definitely associated with food
- reporting only cases of salmonellosis.

In England and Wales food-poisoning cases have been increasing over the last decade so that in 1997 there were approximately 94 000. Of these the most common reported bacterial causes are *Salmonella* and *Campylobacter*. Within the decade to 1997 *Campylobacter* has increased in reported incidence whereas in the last few years at least, *Salmonella* cases have remained relatively stable. There is no evidence that there has been any change in reporting criteria by either clinicians or local laboratories and so this increase seems real (Figure 1.4.).

Figure 1.4. *Salmonella* and *Campylobacter* reports 1987-1997 (from CDSC statistics).

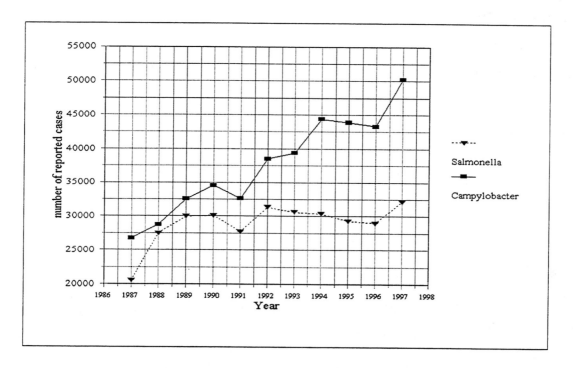

1.6. Why has food-poisoning increased so much?

The food industry spends much of its resources ensuring that the food they provide to the consumer is safe and wholesome. However, the figures of food-poisoning reports are rising at, many would argue, an unacceptable rate. Assuming that these reported rates are a true reflection (as discussed in Section 1.3.) then the increase may be due to a combination of factors:

- changes in shopping habits - shopping less frequently, purchasing larger amounts at each visit resulting in longer periods of storage

- increased public awareness (encouraged by media interest in adverse food scares)

- the increase in the consumer market of chilled ready-prepared foods which have relatively short shelf-lives and require **very** carefully controlled storage temperatures and

15

efficient heating procedures for safety, the need for which the majority of consumers do not fully understand or appreciate

- the emergence of previously unknown micro-organisms or new strains of micro-organisms (Chapter 4)

- increased consumption of so-called 'fast foods' and eating out of the home environment generally.

1.7. Common symptoms

The commonest types of symptom associated with food-poisoning are those related to the gastrointestinal tract including nausea, vomiting, diarrhoea (bloody or otherwise) and abdominal pain. Not all food-associated pathogens necessarily produce all these symptoms and some, such as *Listeria monocytogenes* for example, produce potentially more serious symptoms. The symptoms associated with each pathogen will be described in later chapters.

Toxins produced by the pathogen are generally the means by which the symptoms occur. These toxins may be either **endotoxins** (produced on lysis of the bacterial cell) or **exotoxins** (secreted by the living bacterial cell). Exotoxins may have various mechanisms of action and a particular pathogen may produce more than one type of exotoxin:

- **enterotoxins** which act on mucosal cells lining the gastrointestinal tract (enterocytes) resulting in excessive leakage of fluid from the cell and hence diarrhoea (e.g. *Vibrio cholerae*)

- **cytotoxins** which kill host cells which may result in malfunction of organ systems (e.g. *E. coli* O157 and kidney failure)

- **neurotoxins** which affect nerve cells (e.g. *Clostridium botulinum*).

The symptoms of food-poisoning may be produced by:

- ingestion of a preformed toxin produced in the food by the pathogen (e.g. *Bacillus cereus* or *Staphylococcus aureus*)

- ingestion of a live pathogen which colonises the gastrointestinal tract and produces enterotoxins (e.g. *Clostridium perfringens*)

- ingestion of a live pathogen which invades the cells lining the gut producing inflammation and even ulceration (e.g. *E. coli* (EIEC)).

Vomiting (and the preceding nausea) is the result of stimulation of the vomiting centre in the brain caused by messages from nerve endings in the lining of the gastrointestinal tract. The exact mechanisms are undetermined although activation of these nerve endings is probably due to the direct effect of toxins or because of localised inflammation.

1.8. Who is at risk from food-poisoning?

It is the young, elderly and those immuno-compromised in some way, for example those individuals undergoing radiotherapy or chemotherapy, who are most at risk from all infectious diseases including food-poisoning. Some organisms present a particular risk to other groups such as *Listeria monocytogenes* infection being likely to affect an unborn foetus. Specific risk factors are discussed in more detail in later chapters.

Primary cases are those that initially consumed the contaminated food while secondary cases are those which become infected via person-to-person spread. The latter are the means whereby large outbreaks generally occur and are often of more concern and greater in number than primary cases.

CDSC identified 3499 general outbreaks of infectious intestinal disease in England and Wales between January 1992 and December 1996. Outbreaks are generally associated with the commercial preparation of food served in restaurants, hotels and cafes but do occur via food prepared in a domestic kitchen and served to a number of individuals either in the home or at a function at another location. Although commercial kitchens are submitted to regular inspections and licensing statutes, domestic kitchens have no such control on their hygiene levels. In the two years following the introduction of a new questionnaire by CDSC designed to improve the data collection concerning outbreaks of infectious intestinal disease 642 outbreaks were investigated.

Table 1.5. Settings of general outbreaks of foodborne infectious disease in England and Wales 1992-1994 (compiled from PHLS CDSC statistics).

Setting	Outbreaks (%)
Restaurant, public house, bar	170 (26.5)
Private house	101 (15.7)
Hotel/guest house/residential public house	75 (11.7)
Residential institution	59 (9.2)
Shop / retailer	38 (5.9)
Canteen	35 (5.4)
School	30 (4.7)
Armed services camp	20 (3.1)
Hospital	19 (3.0)
Mobile retailer	5 (0.8)
Other	90 (14.0)
Total	**642 (100.0)**

Restaurants, public houses or bars provided the greatest number of outbreaks with contaminated poultry or eggs being the greatest single cause. However, food prepared at private houses was the setting for 101 of the outbreaks (Table 1. 5.) indicating that public health messages should be addressed to those who prepare food in a domestic setting for consumption by large numbers of individuals. *Salmonella* was the most common organism involved in outbreaks. The factors involved in determining the outbreaks included:

- inappropriate storage
- inadequate heat treatment
- cross contamination
- infected food handler.

Although assessing the cause of each sporadic, i.e. an isolated primary case, is difficult, it is generally accepted that the factors listed above are also risks that apply to the large numbers of non-outbreak cases. Greater public awareness of the risks involved in improper handling, storage and cooking of food will be required before the cases of food-poisoning will decrease to any significant extent.

1.9. Control and prevention of food-poisoning

A variety of codes of practice and laws concerning the processing, handling and sale of foods has been developed at local, national and international levels in order to attempt to protect the public. These have tended to rely on inspectional strategies, supplemented by microbiological testing, even though it is widely acknowledged that both these approaches have serious shortcomings. The food processor generally attempts to comply with relevant laws via in-house quality control procedures including observation of operations and testing physical, chemical and microbiological qualities of the product. Over the last few years a more systematic approach to controlling microbiological hazards has been developed which has been based on the anticipation of hazards associated with the production or use of foods, and the identification of points where the hazards can be controlled.

19

1.9.1. The inspection approach

The laws enforced by EHOs and others involved in the inspection process sometimes contain vague terms that do not specify exactly what comprises compliance. Phrases such as 'cleaned as frequently as necessary', and 'where necessary to prevent introduction of undesirable micro-organisms', may be interpreted differently by different people. The person responsible for compliance with the laws and codes of practice has little or no indication of the relative importance of each specification within the regulations. This means of ensuring food safety relies on a subjective judgement by the inspector who may fail to distinguish between important and not quite so important requirements. Visits to food premises by inspectors are necessarily occasional making their observations restricted in terms of the actual day-to-day operations. The result has been that inspectors rely on the examination of laboratory and process records which may not provide a true reflection of actual events in the premises whether it is a food processing factory, an abattoir or a retail outlet. This approach to the control of microbiological hazards, although limited in terms of effectiveness, does provide a means of control which, if not used, would result in even greater numbers of cases of disease.

1.9.2. Microbiological testing

Microbiological screening is an effective means of assessing whether a product contains human pathogens. Its wide-spread use is relatively recent. Drinking water is an example where such testing has provided an efficient method for protecting public health. However, applying such techniques as a means of controlling microbiological hazards **in foods** is difficult since sufficient representative samples of the product must be obtained in order to collate meaningful information about the microbiological condition of a batch of food. Microbiological methods are time consuming, especially if specific, and are generally expensive. The time involved means that if the product is perishable spoilage might occur while waiting for the results. Also microbiological testing only confirms contamination. It does not identify the source nor does it rectify the problem, making it an inefficient approach to control and prevention.

1.9.3. Hazard analysis

One of the major advances in control and prevention of food-associated illness has been the development of the Hazard Analysis and Critical Control Point (HACCP) philosophy. This is a means whereby 'weak' links in the food chain from 'farm to fork' may be identified. It was first presented in outline form at the 1971 National Conference on Food Protection. It is a systematic approach for applying knowledge of microbiological concepts to the control of the quality of food.

A hazard analysis evaluates all procedures in the production, distribution and use of raw materials and food products, in order to: **identify potentially hazardous raw materials and foods that may contain poisonous substances, pathogens or large numbers of food spoilage micro-organisms, and/or that can support microbial growth.**

Application of hazard analysis allows the concentration of resources in limiting contamination at particular points (critical control points or CCPs) in the food chain which are the most likely to provide means whereby contamination may occur resulting in a hazard to human health. The approach may be applied to all food processing procedures but is particularly applicable to food processing plants and food premises supplying a large number of consumers such as in a home for the elderly or a hospital.

In HACCP language a **hazard** is a source of danger such as the unacceptable growth or survival of a pathogen itself or the production of a toxin by growth or survival of a microbe.

21

A **risk**, on the other hand, is the estimate of the likely occurrence of a hazard. This means that although *Clostridium botulinum* is a much more serious hazard than *Staphylococcus aureus* for example, because its incidence in food has been shown to be relatively much lower it poses a much lower risk. There are many excellent references discussing the HACCP approach in detail and so a brief description only suffices here.

A HACCP programme involves the following stages:

- Hazard analysis
- Identification of critical control points or CCPs
- Establishment of CCP criteria
- Monitoring procedures for CCPs
- Protocols for CCP deviation
- Record keeping
- Verification

Hazard analysis identifies:

- raw materials which **may** contain pathogenic micro-organisms or their toxic metabolites
- points in the process under examination which **might** allow contamination to occur
- stages in the process where microbial growth and survival **may** occur because of the physical or chemical properties of the food
- procedures during the process which, if effectively carried out, **eliminate** hazards i.e. they are bactericidal or bacteriostatic.

1.9.3.1. Critical control points

A CCP is defined as a location, step or procedure at which a level of control can be exercised over a hazard. At a CCP the hazard may be eliminated, prevented or reduced to a defined, acceptable level. Examples of CCPs are shown in Table 1.6.

Table 1.6. Examples of CCPs

Cooking	Heating to 70°C for 2 minutes kills all vegetative cells
Freezing	Most micro-organisms are killed at -20°C: some survive but do not multiply
Refrigeration	Most micro-organisms do not multiply at 4°C but most survive.
Disinfection procedures	Chemicals are available which are effective against most micro-organisms
Staff personal hygiene	Hand-washing reduces significantly contamination
Changes in pH in food	Generally low or high pH reduce multiplication of micro-organisms
Changes in water content of food i.e. drying	All micro-organisms require water for growth and multiplication

1.9.3.2. Monitoring CCPs

At each of the CCPs in a process the criteria must be established by which control will be indicated and limits set for monitoring. For example, if a food is to be refrigerated then the acceptable temperature range must be determined. When these criteria have been agreed then procedures for monitoring should be instituted i.e. at what time intervals will the monitoring take place? If a deviation for the limits set in the criteria are observed then a protocol must be introduced which sets out rectification strategies.

The five main types of monitoring are visual observation, sensory evaluation, physical measurements, chemical testing and microbiological examination. Because the effectiveness of monitoring in terms of CCPs is related directly to the speed with which results are obtained, visual observations are often the most useful. Visual examination of raw materials, cleanliness of plant and equipment, worker hygiene, processing procedures, and storage and transportation facilities are most commonly used. Monitoring procedures chosen must enable action to be taken to rectify an out-of-control situation, either before the start-up, or during the operation of a process. Record-keeping at all stages and at all CCPs is an important part of the HACCP approach. This, together with verification processes, provides a basis for judging the effectiveness of the measures and ensures that the process results in a consistently safe product for the consumer.

1.10. Conclusion

Food safety is an important public health issue and bacteria are a major cause of food-poisoning cases. Proper and effective control of their entry into the human food chain is essential for the reduction in the increasingly large (and, many would argue, unacceptable) number of cases which occur annually in the UK and in other countries. Understanding the environmental reservoirs and vehicles of infection involved means that preventative measures may be put into place which ultimately will fulfil this goal. The following chapters describe the common bacterial causes of food-poisoning and some of the preventative measures instigated by producers, processors and legislators to achieve a reduction in notifications and therefore in human illness caused by bacterial food-borne pathogens.

CHAPTER 2

THE MOST COMMON BACTERIAL FOOD-BORNE PATHOGENS: *CAMPYLOBACTER* AND *SALMONELLA*

2.1. Introduction

The number of reported food-poisoning cases in England and Wales was 94 382 in 1997 which represents an increase of 11% over the previous twelve months figure of 84 423. Two bacteria are responsible for the majority of laboratory confirmed cases. These are *Campylobacter* species which, in England and Wales, was the cause of 50 247 cases in 1997 and *Salmonella* (non-*typhi*) species (32 169 cases in 1997). This chapter describes these bacteria, identifies reasons for the massive increase in their reported incidences over the previous fifteen years, examines the preventative measures, if any, introduced for control and discusses the effectiveness or otherwise of these.

2.2. *Campylobacter* species

Since *Campylobacter jejuni*, the major human pathogen of this genus, was identified in 1977 by Skirrow, it and other campylobacters such as *Campylobacter coli* and *Campylobacter lari* have been recognised as a major public health problem in the UK, USA and many other countries worldwide. *Campylobacter* are Gram-negative, spiral, flagellated rods which are extremely motile and are only able to multiply in low oxygen concentrations.

The genus *Campylobacter* was reclassified in 1994 and now contains seventeen defined species. The main pathogenic campylobacters are *C. jejuni*, *C. coli* and *C. lari* with *C. jejuni* being the most common in the UK, accounting for 90-95% of cases of campylobacter enteritis or campylobacteriosis. *C. jejuni* is further divided into two subspecies: *C. jejuni jejuni* (simply called *C. jejuni*) which is the human pathogen and *C. jejuni doylei* which is very rarely found as the cause of human illness. *C. upsaliensis* is another campylobacter which has been linked with human infection and which is isolated at a high rate from dog faeces. This may therefore be the common cause of *Campylobacter* infection traced to handling of domestic pets but because of the isolation techniques routinely used for detection the true incidence of this organism remains unknown.

2.2.1. *Isolation and detection of Campylobacter*

C. jejuni, *C. coli* and *C. lari* are known as the thermophilic campylobacters because they grow well at temperatures in the range 42-43°C and do not grow below 25°C. Under adverse environmental conditions such as prolonged exposure to water or high oxygen concentrations they change from their spiral rod-like shape to a coccoid form. Their viability in this form is debatable since some workers found that they can colonise the gastrointestinal tract of one-day-old chicks while others dispute this. Certainly the coccoid form cannot be cultured *in vitro* although an antigen characteristic of *Campylobacter* can be detected.

Early attempts to isolate campylobacters from human faeces were based on a membrane filtration method which, with the numbers of investigations undergone in England and Wales in the last few years, is too expensive and resource laden to contemplate as a routine procedure. Presently the organism is isolated from human faecal specimens by incubation at 42-43°C under microaerophilic conditions on selective media especially designed to encourage the growth of *Campylobacter*, specifically the thermophilic campylobacters, **and** discourage the growth of other naturally occurring gut organisms.

The first selective media was developed by Skirrow in 1977 and is still used, with modifications, in clinical laboratories. For veterinary and other environmental specimens the original medium may not be selective enough because of overgrowth of *Campylobacter* by pseudomonads which are common organisms in these types of samples. The similar, but more selective, Preston medium with a pre-enrichment step allows the detection of low numbers of the organism to be detected in food as does the recent blood-free selective media, CAT agar (containing cefoperazone, amphotericin, teicoplanin) and CCDA (cefoperazone, charcoal, deoxycholate agar). However, detection of **very** low numbers may require more sophisticated techniques such as the Latex Agglutination Test (LAT) or Polymerase Chain Reaction (PCR). The latter particularly is an extremely powerful tool in identifying species type.

Until recently the organism was only identified at the genus level and only rarely at species level. Further confirmation and identification using the various biotyping, phage typing and serotyping schemes available to distinguish *Campylobacter* at a more specific level require greater resources than had been previously considered necessary for clinical diagnosis. However, with the increase in number of cases and uncertainty over the means whereby the organism enters and moves within the food chain, the PHLS Laboratory of Enteric Pathogens (LEP) has developed a reference facility for this organism similar to that available for salmonellas. This allows typing to a very specific level and thus, it is hoped, enables clusters of campylobacter infections to be identified and investigated. Heightened surveillance should augment the present knowledge of campylobacter infection and lead to effective preventative measures and control.

2.2.2. Illness caused by Campylobacter

Campylobacter enteritis (or campylobacteriosis) has symptoms which vary between individuals. The incubation time is generally between one and seven days (with an average of three days) and, in the majority of cases, recovery is complete within one week. The symptoms range from those of an asymptomatic illness, characterised fleetingly by loose stools, to abdominal pain, which in extreme cases can be mistakenly diagnosed as acute appendicitis and result in hospitalisation. Bloody diarrhoea with inflammation of the gut lining tends to be common in developed countries, particularly in young adults, whereas in developing counties where infection is endemic, watery stools are a more common symptom and young children are at greater risk. There is also the remote possibility of further serious complications such as Guillain-Barre syndrome (peripheral polyneuritis with severe and sometimes fatal paralysis) and there has also been a report of a spontaneous abortion related to *Campylobacter* (*C. fetus*) infection. The number of organisms required for disease is thought to be as few as 500 cells.

The function of motility in the pathogenesis of campylobacter infection is well established. Motility is required both to enable the organism to reach attachment sites in the intestinal mucosa and to enter epithelial cells. However, the role and even the type of toxin involved in the production of symptoms remains an area of intense investigation currently. *Campylobacter* probably produces enterotoxins and is responsible for the classic symptoms of gastrointestinal disease. However, at least some strains also produce exotoxins such as a hepatotoxin or a cytolethal distending toxin or haemolytic cytotoxin.

The incidence of bacteraemia caused by *Campylobacter* spp., compared with total number of laboratory reports, is very low at approximately 35 per annum. The majority of these are patients over 65 years old with no particular predisposing factors such as underlying disease involved. The reasons for the development of bacteraemia in such patients is undetermined at present.

2.2.3. Epidemiology

Since 1983 *Campylobacter* has been the most common laboratory reported infection in England and Wales. The most important feature of *Campylobacter* epidemiology is the fact that campylobacteriosis almost always occurs as sporadic cases with no secondary spread. This means that each case is a primary one. There are regional and seasonal differences in laboratory reports which complicate the epidemiology of the illness. In 1989-1991 the average rate was 65 cases per 100 000 population with the highest rate being in Yorkshire (approximately 90 per 100 000 population), although above average rates were reported in the Trent, Wessex, Oxford, South West and Wales regions. These figures disguise even more localised high rates. In the North-West region, for example, the rate in Lancaster was 139 per 100 000 in 1989 and 231 in 1990.

Total food-poisoning notifications (both formally notified and otherwise ascertained) usually peak in midsummer (late June to August) and those of *Salmonella* reflect this (Figure 2.3.). However, the reports of *Campylobacter* infection tend to peak earlier, in weeks 25 to 28, i.e. in June. This is a consistent trend observed over several years (Figure 2.1.). In Lancaster this is mirrored by a similar peak in contamination in farm animals but the source of the contamination is, as yet, undetermined. In 1997 over 6500 reports were received by CDSC in weeks 25 to 28 which is the largest number of cases reported in any four-week period to date.

Figure 2.1. Seasonal reports of *Campylobacter* cases (compiled from CDSC data).

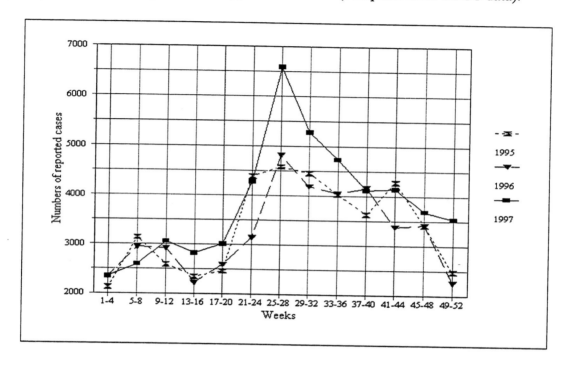

2.2.4. Vehicles of infection

The reasons underlying the seasonal variation in *Campylobacter* infection remain controversial. One factor suggested is the drinking of milk from doorstep delivered bottles which have been pecked by birds. There have been several epidemiological studies suggesting an association between consumption of milk from bottles pecked by birds and *Campylobacter* infection. Crows and magpies have been photographed pecking milk bottles which have been subsequently proved to contain the organism. Birds have a higher body temperature than humans (approximately 42°C) which would make them ideal for providing an environmental reservoir. Crows and magpies are scavengers and, by pecking their own faeces and those of other animals, they can act as vectors for the transmission of *Campylobacter* into the human food chain. Although there have been many public health warnings against consumption of bird-pecked milk recent studies still suggest that consumers are either unaware of the health risks involved or choose to ignore them. However this source may be the cause of the seasonal rise in campylobacter infections (pecking of milk by birds increases in May-June possibly because of feeding of young) but it cannot account for the large increase in laboratory reports over the last decade since doorstep milk deliveries have dramatically decreased over a similar period (Figure 2.2.), although total sales have remained at approximately 5800 million litres per annum.

Figure 2.2. Percentage of milk which is delivered to doorstep in UK.

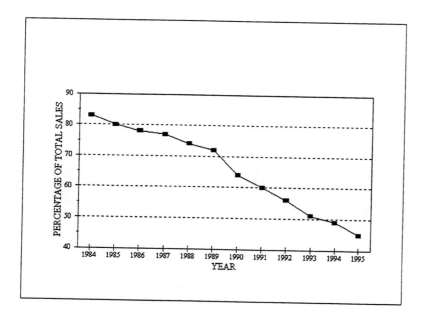

In 1993 a report by the Advisory Committee for Microbiological Safety of Food suggested that this may be such a potential cause of campylobacter infection that milk bottle tops should be redesigned but to date, no progress has been made in this important area of public health.

The organism is not able to survive proper pasteurisation procedures but raw milk may be a source of infection and there have been several reports of cases linked to the consumption of raw milk by children after educational visits to farms. Post-pasteurisation contamination at the dairy has also been the cause of some outbreaks.

However, outbreaks of campylobacter infection are relatively rare events especially considering the fact that the pathogen itself is so common. Only 240 (0.2%) of 122 250 cases of campylobacteriosis reported between 1992 and 1994 were associated with general outbreaks, of which there were twenty-one. Vehicles of infection were identified in sixteen of these outbreaks with eight food-borne, four caused by milk and five water-borne. Extensive studies of sporadic illness by the PHLS has indicated that handling and preparation of raw meat, exposure to pets with diarrhoea, ingestion of raw milk or milk from bottles with tops pecked by birds or untreated water are major risk factors for infection. However, occupational exposure to live animals or faecal samples (through farming, microbiology or veterinary or medical practice) or handling of whole chickens with giblets in a domestic environment or eating a dish prepared from the chicken brought into the home in this way seems to **decrease** the risk for developing infection. This suggests that continuous exposure results in a certain degree of immunity.

Since *Campylobacter* are normal inhabitants of the intestinal tract of a wide range of birds and mammals, contamination of meat occurs from the gut to the meat during processing at the abattoir. Although the organism may not be able to grow during the post-processing period because of efficient chilling, they are able to survive. Surveys of poultry suggest that between 30% and 100% of all broilers on retail sale may be contaminated by *Campylobacter*. Pork has also been shown to be contaminated at the abattoir and approximately 10% of pork carcasses in the USA are infected. Cross contamination has been shown to be an important way in which the organism can enter the human food chain. Storage of contaminated poultry close to other food products which do not undergo subsequent cooking such as salad vegetables or the use of the same (or unwashed) chopping board and/or knife for the preparation of raw meat and food which is consumed uncooked results in a risk of infection. However, although poultry is a major source of human infection, eggs are not generally contaminated by *Campylobacter*.

2.2.5. Treatment

Campylobacter infections are self-limiting and do not require anti-microbial treatment. However, in severe cases or those of particularly susceptible groups, such as very young infants, medical advice should be sought. Most isolates are sensitive to a wide range of antibiotics. Erythromycin is the drug of first choice because of its low toxicity and narrow spectrum of activity although its clinical effectiveness is doubtful. If this is contraindicated then fluoroquinolones are a safe, effective but expensive alternative.

2.3. *Salmonella* species

Almost all salmonellas are able to cause human disease. The most severe illness caused by *Salmonella* species is typhoid which is the result of infection by *S. typhi* and *S. paratyphi*. This disease, which, although it is a gastrointestinal infectious illness, is also notifiable in its own right. It is an enteric fever and, as such, is outside the scope of this book.

Salmonella are Gram-negative, flagellated rod-shaped bacteria which, unlike *Campylobacter*, are able to grow under a wide range of conditions. They multiply both in aerobic and anaerobic situations and within a pH range of 4 to 8. They are resistant to freezing and drying but are killed by heat (71.7°C for 15 seconds) and acids below pH4.

Until the early 1980s *S. typhimurium* was the most commonly isolated salmonella in England and Wales accounting for 51% (7785 out of a total of 15 155 cases) in 1983. Since then there has been a massive increase in the numbers of cases caused by *S. enteritidis* so that in 1997 14% of the cases were *S. typhimurium* and 71% *S. enteritidis* (4645 and 22 806 cases respectively).

2.3.1. Isolation and detection

Salmonella are classified according to the Kauffmann-White scheme which divides them into over 2000 serotypes depending on the somatic (O), flagella (H) and capsular (Vi) antigens present. For epidemiological studies a more discriminative method of distinguishing salmonellas has been utilised by the PHLS using phage typing. This is where each isolate is subjected to infection by a set of phages (bacterial viruses) and then classified according to which phage type it is susceptible. In the case of *S. enteritidis,* phage type 4 (PT4) represents the vast majority of isolates in England and Wales but PT8 and PT13a in the USA. The most common type of *S. typhimurium* is DT 104. The organisms may be easily isolated from faeces of suspected cases and also from food vehicles by conventional culturing procedures such as pre-enrichment in selenite-cystine or Rappaport-Vassiliadis broth followed respectively by incubation on bismuth-sulphite agar or brilliant green modified agar. Characteristic colonies may be confirmed as *Salmonella* by biochemical tests.

2.3.2. Illness caused by Salmonella

The main symptoms of *Salmonella* enteritis are nausea, vomiting, diarrhoea, abdominal pain, fever and chills. General malaise, headaches and loss of weight and appetite may also occur. The incubation period is 5-72 hours but may be as long as seven days with symptoms occurring between 12 and 36 hours after infection and lasting two to five days. The severity of the illness depends on various factors:

- whether the person infected is particularly susceptible (i.e. the elderly or very young)
- the number of cells ingested
- the food vehicle involved.

The infective dose is usually one million cells but if the food vehicle contains a high fat content such as chocolate or cheese then it may be as low as ten cells particularly if susceptible individuals are involved. It has been suggested that the high fat content somehow protects the organism from the acid stomach environment allowing a more efficient colonisation of the intestinal mucosa. The death rate from salmonellosis is higher than that from other food-borne disease especially in the elderly and those that have an underlying disease such as AIDS or cancer. Damage to the mucosal cells lining the intestine may result in long-term problems with improper nutrient absorption and hence malnutrition. This increases the risk of development of allergies such as irritable bowel syndrome (IBS).

2.3.3. *Epidemiology*

The number of cases of *Salmonella* infection has not mirrored the rise in *Campylobacter* infections. For the years 1995-7 the numbers have remained fairly constant. The annual peak in incidence is related to that of total food poisoning incidents and occurs in summer (Figure 2.3). This has been attributed to the rise in temperatures usually experienced at this time of year and the increase in *al fresco*-type meals such as picnics and barbecues. There is a statistically significant relationship between monthly temperature and reported cases of food-poisoning (and therefore *Salmonella* infection) in that month. However, there is also a relationship between monthly reports and the temperature in the **previous** month. This suggests that infection does not only occur at point of consumption but also earlier in the food chain such as in the abattoir and during subsequent processing.

Figure 2.3. Seasonal reported food poisoning notifications and *Salmonella* cases.

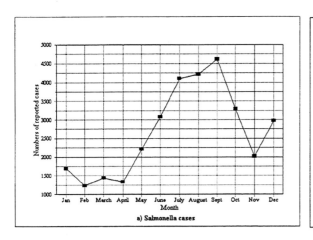

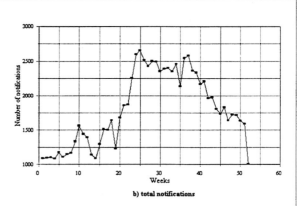

Salmonella species account for the majority of the general outbreaks reported in England and Wales (Table 2.1.).

Table 2.1. Pathogens identified in general outbreaks of food-borne infectious intestinal disease in England and Wales 1992-4 (compiled from CDSC data).

Pathogen	Number of outbreaks (%)
S. enteritidis PT4	239 (37.2)
other *S. enteritidis*	40 (6.2)
S. typhimurium	52 (8.1)
S. virchow	11 (1.7)
other *Salmonella* serotypes	20 (3.1)
other identified organisms	200 (31.2)
unknown	80 (12.5)
Total	642 (100)

2.3.4. *Vehicles of infection*

Salmonella are often present in the gastrointestinal tract of poultry and other animals. Primary infection of humans occurs by consumption of contaminated food or water. Secondary infections are common with the faecal-oral route being the most frequent means of spread between individuals.

Within the farm environment animals including poultry may become infected by a number of different routes (Figure 2.4.) which has resulted in widespread infection of commercial poultry flocks. Vertical transmission results in infection passing from breeding flocks to layers.

Figure 2.4. Transmission routes of *Salmonella* (Baird-Parker,1990, *The Lancet*: reproduced with permission).

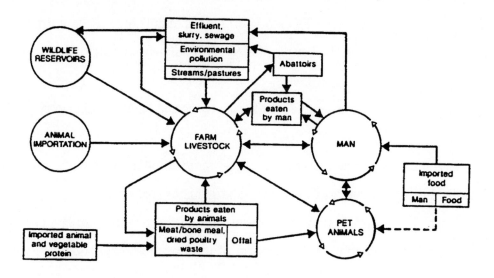

Poultry on retail sale is frequently contaminated with *Salmonella*. Some studies have reported a contamination rate of over 60%. Risk of infection is high if the contaminated poultry is either eaten raw, undercooked or mishandled after cooking (when cross-contamination can occur) and then held for several hours. Cooked turkey meat is a common source of *Salmonella* since turkeys tend to be large products which require a long time to thaw, cook, cool and reheat. This gives many opportunities for mishandling, inadequate cooking or improper storage. Processing of raw poultry meat such as deboning, grinding or chopping provides a means by which cross contamination may occur via food preparation surfaces, utensils and hands.

The bacterium reaches the tissues via the circulation **after** death during post-slaughter processing. When the chicken is dipped in the scalding water-bath after slaughter the heart is still beating thus allowing distribution to the tissues. Ascending infection spreading from the cloaca may also provide a means of reproductive tract and hence egg contamination before the shell is formed. Eggs may also be infected through the shell either as the egg passes down the oviduct or immediately after laying when the immature cuticle appears to be an ineffective barrier from the surrounding environment in which faeces are common.

The large increase in the number of *Salmonella* reports over recent years has been mainly due to the increase in *S. enteritidis,* especially PT4 serotype. This is mainly associated with eggs, egg products and poultry (particularly chicken) while *S. typhimurium,* although associated with chicken, is also a contaminant of other meats. Food vehicles associated with outbreaks of *S. typhimurium* infection include: unpasteurised milk, meat pies and pasties and bakery products.

Evidence from natural and experimental infections has indicated that some eggs produced by infected hens probably only contain small numbers of organisms (probably ten or less), usually in the white of the egg. Inappropriate storage results in multiplication within the egg, particularly the yolk, so that the recommendation by Department of Health is that eggs should be stored at refrigeration temperatures. Mishandling during the preparation of egg dishes, particularly those which receive little or no subsequent cooking, e.g. mousse has been shown to be a major factor in many outbreaks.

In 1991 the PHLS reported on a survey carried out on eggs (both produced in the UK and imported) which found that the risk of contamination from *S. enteritidis* PT4 was about one in 1320 for UK eggs and one in 3040 for imported eggs. The survey did not differentiate between organisms found inside the egg or those on the shell and concluded that the risk to the individual from consuming a single egg was very low. However, since some ten billion eggs are produced annually in the UK there must be a substantial number of eggs on sale which are contaminated with *S. enteritidis*. The massive programme of eradication begun in the late 1980s by MAFF and the egg industry resulted in large numbers of layers and pullets being destroyed and the adoption of the EC Zoonoses Directive in 1993 seeks to reduce vertical transmission from breeding flocks to layers. However, complete eradication is still a long way from being realised.

Despite the Department of Health advice published in 1988 concerning the risk from consuming raw eggs and raw egg dishes particularly by the young, the elderly the sick and pregnant mothers, sporadic cases and outbreaks are still caused by this source. Salmonellas are able to survive cooking in situations when the yolk remains liquid. Provided that the number of cells of *S. enteritidis* PT4 initially present in the egg before cooking is less than $\log_{10} 8.0$ per gram, the organism is eliminated by scrambling rapidly at high temperatures, boiling for nine minutes or longer or frying 'over easy' until all the yolk had solidified. With scrambled eggs reaching a temperature of 80°C in the cooked mix is important.

Mayonnaise, tiramisu and mousses, all of which use raw egg in their preparation and are not cooked, have been commonly associated with cases. In 1995 there was an outbreak caused by consumption of marshmallow confectionry from a bakery which affected several people, mainly children. The use of pasteurised egg should have become embedded in commercial and domestic procedures but it appears that, after the initial heeding of the 1988 warning and because of the media interest in other food-associated pathogens, some caterers and others are assuming eggs are no longer a problem.

The effectiveness of the surveillance scheme of the PHLS for salmonellas (Salm-Net) towards identifying outbreaks and their source resulting in a halting of a risk of infection to a large number of individuals has recently been reported. Between 5th December 1994 and 30th January 1995 27 cases of infection by *S. agona* PT15 were identified in England and Wales. Case-control analysis of the food habits of those infected (26 of whom were children) indicated that consumption of a kosher savoury snack imported from Israel was strongly linked to illness. Examination of samples of the snack resulted in isolation of *S. agona* PT15. International links with USA, Canada and Israel allowed more cases to be identified and also correlated with consumption of the same snack which was found to have been manufactured on at least seven different dates in a four month period. The product was recalled and the infection controlled. This was an unusual outbreak but it showed how communication between public health authorities in different countries is important when attempting to investigate such cases.

Poultry is not the only meat contaminated with salmonellas. Surveys of pig meat both in the UK and USA suggest that anywhere between 5% and 40% (depending on source) of pig carcasses leaving the abattoir and entering the human food chain are contaminated with this organism. Beef and lamb carcasses have a much lower rate of contamination at approximately 1%. *S. typhimurium* is the most common salmonella found in these types of meat and meat products but, at the present, *S. enteritidis* infections are the most important in terms of numbers in England and Wales.

2.3.5. Treatment

Treatment of salmonellosis is by fluid replacement therapy since treatment with antibiotics generally results in a prolongation of the carrier state. In those cases without complications therefore this is the best method of treatment.

2.4. Control and prevention of *Campylobacter* and *Salmonella*

Both these organisms are common contaminants of fresh meat, particularly poultry. *Campylobacter* is also frequently present in raw milk while raw eggs often contain *Salmonella*. Effective cooking or pasteurisation procedures eliminate both organisms so that some reasons that human infection occurs may be:

- consumption of undercooked food containing the organism

- post cooking contamination of the food in question

- cross contamination by primary infected food to food which is to be consumed without further (or any) cooking.

Although the media has stimulated interest and awareness in the general population on this topic, the numbers of cases continue to rise. Therefore, proper education is an essential part of the task of reducing food-poisoning cases. There are various ways in which the primary infection rate may be reduced since if the food entering the food chain is relatively free of organisms the likelihood of infection occurring further up the chain will be reduced.

2.4.1. At the farm

At the farm strict hygiene procedures will reduce infection of animals while, for the future, vaccines may be the only way that the organisms will be eliminated from the breeding and laying flocks. Competitive exclusion techniques can be used to prevent colonisation of chicks by pathogenic organisms. These techniques involve the introduction of a specific cocktail of micro-organisms into the caecum of one-day-old chicks. This cocktail is rigorously selected from the caecum of adult birds so that the micro-organisms can specifically compete for the 'niche' in the gastrointestinal tract which may have been occupied by salmonellas or campylobacters thus

41

preventing colonisation by the pathogen. Exclusion techniques may provide a less expensive but just as effective method of control as vaccines.

Animal feed may also be a source of pathogens because the raw materials used to make meat and bone meal were themselves contaminated (Figure 2.4.). Although the process of 'hot pelleting' (extrusion of hot mash under pressure to form pellets) destroys any bacteria present post-processing contamination results in at least some animal feed containing salmonellas. The farming community are notoriously slow in instigating any procedures it considers might reduce their profit margin but eventually complete eradication at the farm may be the only way to protect the consumer.

2.4.2. At the abattoir

Transportation to the abattoir under crowded or otherwise stressful conditions provides an opportunity for cross infection since the excretion of the organisms in the faeces will increase in these circumstances. At the abattoir itself there are many stages in the process such as slaughter, dressing and preparation of raw meat at which contamination might (and does) occur. The skins of animals may have high counts of pathogenic bacteria as do, of course, intestinal contents which may contaminate muscle during the gutting process. The use of mechanical eviscerators in poultry plants means that, from time to time, an intestinal tract becomes ruptured thus contaminating a potentially large number of carcasses which subsequentially pass through the machine before cleaning. Raw meat entering the human food chain frequently therefore contains pathogenic organisms and this is particularly the case for salmonellas and campylobacters.

Post-slaughter washes have been suggested as an effective means of reducing contamination. Trisodium phosphate (TSP) is approved by the US government as a post-chill anti-microbial agent for raw poultry meat. Treatment with TSP reduces the populations of *C. jejuni* and *S.*

typhimurium, does not affect taste or texture of poultry meat and increases the shelf life of the product. Other washes tested include lactic acid and lactic acid/sodium lactate buffer which have also been shown to reduce pathogenic contamination.

Another control method is the use of efficient post-slaughter chilling procedures which reduce the survival and growth of both *Campylobacter* spp. and *Salmonella* spp. but this must be continuously maintained at all stages of processing and storage. A combination of post-slaughter washes and chilling procedures probably provide the most satisfactory and effective method of ensuring the delivery of safe food to the consumer, although irradiation techniques (Chapter 5) are also very effective in controlling levels of pathogens. At the present time, however, the public's attitude towards irradiated foods is one of suspicion and ambivalence.

2.4.3. Food processors and retailers

The legal responsibility of the food industry overall will be discussed in detail in Chapter 6. Suffice it to mention here that at all stages of the preparation and storage of food products, use of the HACCP approach (Chapter 1) will decrease the risk of food-borne illness. The maintenance of the 'chill chain', i.e. the storage of foods at appropriate temperatures during transportation and retail display which reduces survival and multiplication of pathogens is essential for food safety.

2.4.4. In the kitchen

Commercial kitchen hygiene is under the control of legislation and such premises are subjected to regular inspections by EHOs. The adherence to the legal requirements is the responsibility of the person in charge. However, as has been previously discussed in Chapter 1, food prepared in the domestic kitchen causes many outbreaks. To reduce or even eliminate the risk of food poisoning by all pathogens but particularly campylobacters and salmonellas because of their prevalence in raw meat several good practices must be instituted in the domestic kitchen:

- storage at correct temperature
- separate storage of cooked and raw food or at least within a storage facility cooked food stored above raw food rather than vice versa
- use of different chopping boards for raw meat and other foods
- good personal hygiene, e.g. hand washing
- thorough reheating (including microwaving) of previously cooked food whether bought ready-to-eat or cooked earlier
- use of effective disinfection procedures for cleaning of food preparation surfaces
- regular washing of any cleaning cloths used.

In the final analysis it is only by education of the community at large will the incidence of food poisoning in general and therefore that caused by these two bacteria be reduced. Risky practices should be brought to the attention of the public and awareness of the scope of the problem emphasised. Recent suggested legislation (Chapter 6) in the UK attempts to address this issue and only time will tell how successful it will be.

CHAPTER 3

LESS COMMON BACTERIAL FOOD-BORNE PATHOGENS

3.1. Introduction

Although *Salmonella* spp. and *Campylobacter* spp. cause most of the cases of food-poisoning (Table 3.1.) several other types of bacteria contribute to the overall total of cases. Some of these are important because of the severity of the symptoms they cause, for example *Clostridium botulinum,* or because of the fact that they are able to grow in temperatures at which other bacteria are not able to multiply, for example *Listeria monocytogenes.*

This chapter describes these less common causes of bacterial food poisoning. For each organism, the illness they produce, methods used for their detection and isolation, their epidemiology, the vehicles of infection involved and treatment is outlined.

Table 3.1. Comparison of numbers of cases of bacterial food-poisoning in England and Wales 1986-1996 (data from PHLS Communicable Disease Surveillance Centre).

Year	Total	*Salmonella* spp.	*Campylobacter*	*Bacillus*	*Clostridium perfringens*	*Listeria monocytogenes*	*Staph. aureus*
1986	23 940	16 976	24 110	65	896	129	76
1987	29 331	20 532	26 750	137	1266	238	178
1988	39 713	27 478	28 761	418	1312	278	111
1989	52 557	29 998	32 526	164	901	237	104
1990	52 145	30 112	34 552	162	1442	116	55
1991	52 543	27 693	32 636	95	733	127	61
1992	63 347	31 355	38 552	182	805	106	112
1993	68 587	30 650	39 422	31	562	102	28
1994	81 833	30 411	44 414	87	449	112	74
1995	82 041	29 314	43 876	87	342	85	59
1996	83 233	28 983	43 337	27	720	115	150

3.2. *Aeromonas*

These organisms are Gram-negative, facultatively anaerobic, non-spore forming bacilli of which three species (*A. hydrophila, A. sobria, A. caviae)* are confirmed pathogens in children. However, there is controversy concerning their pathogenicity in adults. Some studies have indicated *Aeromonas* as the sole apparent pathogen in acute adult diarrhoea in several areas with a negligible asymptomatic carriage rate, thus lending support to the idea that it may be an enteropathogen in adults. In 1991, the first case of human intestinal *Aeromonas* infection was reported, where the food source was identified as contaminated shellfish. The most important feature of this species, especially *A. hydrophila,* is the fact that the organism is able to survive and multiply at low temperatures (as low as -0.1°C in some strains).

46

3.2.1. Isolation

Direct plating techniques are usually effective in isolating the organism especially where high numbers are present such as in faeces. Starch-ampicillin agar (SA) is the optimal medium for selectivity and differentiation for *Aeromonas* spp. Other media suggested for isolation from faeces include brilliant green bile agar and xylose desoxycholate citrate agar (XDCA). For isolation from environmental samples, pre-enrichment in either alkaline peptone water or trypticase soy-ampicillin broth may be required. Further biochemical tests, particularly the oxidase test, are required for discrimination from *Escherichia coli* and *Klebsiella* spp. An *Aeromonas* serotyping scheme is now available to aid identification in the event of an outbreak.

3.2.2. Illness

Aeromonas poisoning results in profuse watery diarrhoea of one to seven days' duration that is mild and self-limiting. It occurs most commonly in children of less than five years old when the symptoms may be more severe than in infected adults. Other symptoms include abdominal pain, chills and headaches, nausea and colitis. There have been cases where symptoms have lasted for several weeks. As yet, the actual mechanism by which this organism produces these symptoms is undetermined but *A. hydrophila* is generally thought to produce a proteinaceous enterotoxin together with a haemolysin and possibly a cytotoxin. Other virulence factors, related to the way in which the organism colonises the gut, are also important in pathogenesis.

3.2.3. Epidemiology

A. hydrophila food poisoning occurs sporadically rather than in outbreaks. This may reflect surveillance regimes rather than actuality. The infective dose is not known but may be as large as 10^9 cells. Most concern is associated with the consumption of food or water containing this organism by immuno-suppressed or compromised individuals such as cancer patients undergoing therapy or those with AIDS.

3.2.4. Vehicles of infection

Traditionally *Aeromonas* spp. have been considered water-borne pathogens since water is a well-established vehicle for infection. It may be a cause of "travellers' diarrhoea" in some geographical areas such as Thailand where endemic infection is high and where travellers reporting symptoms have a higher incidence than unaffected individuals. However, *A. hydrophila* has been isolated from a wide range of foods such as chilled meats, fish and poultry, raw milk and salad vegetables. Its ability to survive and multiply at refrigerator temperatures means that foods stored for some time under these conditions may contain enough of an infective dose to cause illness. It has been reported that *A. hydrophila* is able to increase in numbers by ten to a thousand fold in meat and fish stored for one week at 4°C.

3.2.5. Treatment

The symptoms are usually self-limiting and anti-microbial treatment is not required. Rarely, cholera-like symptoms occur, when the patient will require rehydration and/or antibiotic therapy.

3.3. *Bacillus cereus*

These are Gram-positive, facultatively anaerobic, endospore-forming organisms that have been known as an agent of food poisoning for many years. However, it is only recently that two different syndromes have been recognized, each caused by a different toxin: the emetic that is heat-stable and the diarrhoeal that is heat sensitive.

3.3.1. *Isolation and detection*

Generally food vehicles of *B. cereus* poisoning contain large numbers of organisms as do faeces and other clinical specimens and so enrichment techniques are not required for isolation. Incubation on a blood-based agar for 24 hours at 37°C is sufficient for most samples. However, there are selective media such as PEMBA (polymyxin/pyruvate/egg yolk/mannitol) for use for secondary confirmation or when numbers of contaminants are low. The heat-labile diarrhoeal toxin can be detected by a sensitive latex agglutination test that is commercially available but neither toxin detection nor serotyping are used routinely in surveillance.

3.3.2. *Illness*

The emetic disease follows the ingestion of a toxin that is a heat-stable protein associated with, or produced during, spore formation. Symptoms often resemble staphylococcal food-poisoning, with a rapid onset of nausea, vomiting and malaise, usually within one to six hours after consumption of the contaminated food, and similarly complications are rare and recovery

49

complete within 24 hours.

The diarrhoeal disease symptoms of profuse watery diarrhoea and abdominal pain resemble those caused by *Clostridium perfringens* with the onset between eight and sixteen hours after consumption of contaminated food and lasting between twelve and 24 hours. In the diarrhoeal syndrome nausea and vomiting are not common but may occur. The toxin involved is thought to be produced in the gastrointestinal tract but may also be produced in the food before consumption.

3.3.3. Epidemiology

In the UK and the USA, the incidence of *B. cereus* food-poisoning is not particularly high in comparison with those caused by *Salmonella* and *Campylobacter*. The emetic type of disease is usually associated with rice and fried rice and many outbreaks have occurred in restaurants serving oriental foods. In the 1970s, of the 110 reported incidents of emetic *B. cereus* food poisoning in the UK, all but two were associated with rice, usually in the form of Chinese fried-rice dishes. Another Bacillus species *B. subtilis*, has also been implicated as a cause of the emetic syndrome with a particularly rapid onset. It is assumed that the toxin produced by this organism is similar to that of *B. cereus*. *B. subtilis* food poisoning has been associated mainly with meat and pastry dishes.

The diarrhoeal syndrome has been associated with consumption of a wide range of foods such as meat products, vegetables, soups and sauces.

3.3.4. Vehicles of infection

Since Bacillus species are ubiquitous in the environment, these organisms will almost always contaminate food and may be found in large numbers in natural, domestic and hospital environments. It is only when large numbers of organisms are present or when they produce the toxin that *B. cereus* becomes a hazard. Commonly the inadequate reheating of food causes outbreaks associated with toxin production.

In outbreaks associated with Chinese 'take-away' dishes, toxin production follows inadequate cooking and proper storage. *B. cereus* spores, which occur commonly in rice, can be relatively heat resistant and so are not always killed during the initial cooking process. The heating process itself selects for spores of greater heat resistance. When the rice cools, and if it is not stored below 8°C, spore germination occurs resulting in vegetative cell growth that may be rapid. Some vegetative cells may sporulate leading to toxin formation, especially if the rice is left for more than a few hours in a fairly warm atmosphere. Although the rice may be further cooked, e.g. fried before serving, the toxin is heat stable and can withstand exposure at 120°C for ninety minutes.

For proper control of *B. cereus* food-poisoning rice should not be reheated after cooking, or, if this is not possible, rapid cooling and final refrigeration of the product should occur.

3.3.5. Treatment

Symptoms caused by *B. cereus* are self-limiting and do not generally require anti-microbial treatment. However, in severe cases rehydration therapy may be necessary.

3.4. *Clostridium botulinum*

Cl. botulinum is a Gram-positive, obligate anaerobe that forms heat resistant spores. It is a common contaminant of soil although it is sometimes found in the gastrointestinal tract of birds and mammals. It grows at a wide range of pHs (4-8.9) and is inhibited at low temperatures. Growth (and therefore toxin production) has been reported in vacuum packaged fish at temperatures as low as 5°C after fifteen days' storage. In other food products the organism may not grow for considerable time (one to three months), especially at the lower temperature of 3.3°C, but this depends on the type of food involved and the initial inoculum.

3.4.1. Isolation and detection

Identification of the organism is based on the ability of a particular colony to produce a toxin. Since the organism may only be a small proportion of the total microflora present, pre-enrichment in cooked meat broth for seven days, followed by anaerobic incubation at 37°C for three days on horse-blood or egg-yolk agar is recommended. A range of *in vitro* immunoassays have been developed for the detection of toxin-producing colonies. The most sensitive method is an *in vivo* method using mice. However, this is becoming increasingly replaced because of the nature of the test.

3.4.2. Illness

Botulism is a serious disease with a mortality rate of between 20% and 50%. It is caused by the consumption of *Cl. botulinum* toxins produced as exotoxins during the growth of *Cl. botulinum* in food. These are neurotoxins and are the most potent natural poisons known. The lethal dose for an adult is about 10^{-8}g. Eight different toxin types have been characterised although botulism in man is usually caused by types A, B and E, and more rarely F and G. Once the toxin is absorbed, it attaches to the neuromuscular junction of affected nerves and prevents the release of the neurotransmitter acetylcholine resulting in muscular paralysis.

The first symptoms of botulism usually develop between twelve and forty-eight hours after consumption of contaminated food but may be as long as eight days. Symptoms may differ, depending on the causative *Cl. botulinum* type, and may include dizziness, difficulty in swallowing, slurred speech, weakness of limbs and blurred vision so that early detection, essential for effective treatment, may not occur. Vomiting and diarrhoea may be reported but there is usually no fever. Breathing problems caused by respiratory paralysis may result in death by asphyxiation.

3.4.3. Epidemiology

Food-borne botulism is a disease that is infrequent in the UK. An outbreak was recorded in 1989 involving twenty-seven patients when nut puree added to yoghurt was contaminated with the organism. Most cases traditionally have been associated with consumption of faultily processed canned food. This is because the cans allow any surviving spores from the heating process to germinate and produce toxins. Home canned and bottled fruit and vegetables were also major contributors to the overall number of cases previously. However, cases of botulism have been declining worldwide over the years, especially in the developed countries where the food manufacturers have applied HACCP principles to their processes in order to eliminate *Cl. botulinum* from the human food chain. Also home preserving of food has also declined, mainly for social reasons.

Infant botulism is different from typical botulism in that it is caused by *Cl. botulinum* producing toxins *in vivo* in the gut. It occurs in infants between two weeks and six months old and is related to the introduction into the diet of 'solid', i.e. non milk-based, foods. Ingestion of a very small number of organisms or spores results in illness because the gut microflora is not well-developed at this stage and cannot out-compete *Cl. botulinum*. It is a very rare disease indeed in the UK but more common in the USA where some cases have been related to the ingestion of honey, presumably containing spores of the organism.

3.4.4. Vehicles of infection

Cl. botulinum may be found in soil and mud, from where it is easily isolated. Since *Cl. botulinum* is strictly anaerobic, botulism is only associated with foods that provide suitable anaerobic conditions. In addition *Cl. botulinum* spores are heat resistant and are able to survive treatment for two hours in boiling water. They are only inactivated during proper food processing procedures that have been carefully researched by the food processing industry (particularly the canning industry) and even more thoroughly monitored. If the parameters are not strictly maintained, *Cl. botulinum* spores may germinate allowing vegetative cells to emerge and toxin production to occur.

Historically, botulism has been associated with home-preserved foods and vegetables but now the disease is mainly associated with improperly processed canned meats and traditional fermented foods such as those made with contaminated vegetables. These often show no obvious signs of spoilage and therefore the consumer is unaware of the contamination before consumption.

Food treatments designed to reduce the growth of the organism rather than eliminate it involve

54

controlling one or more of the following factors in the food: pH, a_w (water activity), temperature, salt concentration, Eh (redox potential), preservative concentration (e.g. nitrite) and oxygen. Although a number of preserved foods are potentially hazardous, growth of *Cl. botulinum* and toxin production usually occur because of faulty manufacturing conditions or through storage at the incorrect temperature. However, since boiling destroys the toxin in a few minutes, adequate cooking before consumption will render contaminated food harmless.

3.4.5. Treatment

Survival is very much dependant on early diagnosis since little can be done to alleviate the effects of any toxin already affecting the neuromuscular junction. However, neuromuscular blocking agents such as 4-aminopyridine may produce transient improvement in symptoms. Timely treatment involves washing the stomach free of any remaining toxic food, intravenous administration of antitoxins and respiratory support, if required.

3.5. Clostridium perfringens

Clostridium perfringens, formerly known as *Cl. welchii*, has been the recognised cause of gas gangrene for over one hundred years. The species consists of Gram-positive, obligate anaerobic, endospore-forming rod-shaped organisms of which there are five major types (A-E) classified according to the number and type of toxin produced. *Cl. perfringens* type A is the cause of both food-poisoning and gas gangrene.

The spores vary in their heat resistance but most food-poisoning outbreaks are caused by those that are the more heat resistant. The enterotoxin is heat-sensitive and its production is intimately involved in spore formation.

3.5.1. Isolation and detection

Cl. perfringens is easy to isolate from clinical and environmental samples because its rapid growth rate ensures that it is present in high numbers in contaminated foods and clinical samples. Incubation anaerobically for 24 hours at 37°C on tryptose-sulphite-cycloserine (TSC) agar either with or without egg yolk, on which *Cl. perfringens* forms black colonies, provides the best available medium for isolation and enumeration. The absence of motility as well as various biochemical tests can be used to further confirm identity. Serotyping based on capsular antigens is used in epidemiological studies of food-poisoning outbreaks. It is also useful in identifying the source of wound infection, i.e. environmental or the bowel of the patient or dressings of the wound.

A number of techniques are available for detecting enterotoxin in clinical and food samples. These include ELISA and latex agglutination tests as well as a biological assay using the rate of killing of Vero cells *in vitro*. DNA probes have also been used to detect *Cl. perfringens* strains that have the ability to produce enterotoxin.

3.5.2. Illness

The symptoms of *Cl. perfringens* food-poisoning are abdominal pain, nausea and acute diarrhoea usually 8-24 hours after the ingestion of food contaminated with large numbers of organisms. Recovery is usually complete within two days. The symptoms are the result of some ingested cells surviving the acid conditions of the stomach and colonising the small intestine where they grow and produce spores and hence enterotoxin. The enterotoxin then binds to proteins on the surface of gut epithelial cells altering various characteristics of the biochemistry of the cell resulting in cell death and thus clinical symptoms.

3.5.3. Epidemiology

The majority of cases of food-poisoning caused by *Cl. perfringens* each year in England and Wales occur in outbreaks with only thirty-five sporadic cases occurring between 1986 and 1996. In this period there was a total of 454 outbreaks totalling 9428 cases. There was a decrease in reported cases between 1992 and 1995 but this trend has not been sustained (Table 3.1.). Outbreaks of *Cl. perfringens* food-poisoning do not seem to have a seasonal incidence and occur throughout the year. They are generally related to preparation of food for large numbers of people where cooking is followed by long periods of storage at abusive temperatures thus allowing the multiplication of the organism to levels that are able to cause illness.

3.5.4. Vehicles of infection

When contaminated food (typically meat) is cooked, anaerobic conditions develop which induces sporulation of the bacteria. When the food is subsequentially cooled, germination of the spores occurs and the resulting vegetative cells continue to multiply, unless the meat is cooled rapidly and kept refrigerated until being reheated thoroughly before consumption. *Cl. perfringens* is able to proliferate over a wide temperature range (15-50°C) with an optimal growth rate occurring at between 43°C and 47°C, when the population may double in as little time as twelve minutes which means that **rapid** cooling is essential to reduce risk.

Enteritis necroticans ('pig-bel') is a rare disease related to *Cl. perfringens* type C strains. It has been reported in Germany and Papua New Guinea. It is caused by the presence of substances in food that are heat-stable trypsin inhibitors that prevent the destruction of the toxin produced by type C strains. This toxin is responsible for the resulting necrotic condition which may be fatal. Profuse watery diarrhoea results in contamination of the environments and hence animals. Pigs seem to be particularly susceptible to infection. The dietary combination of contaminated pork, especially pork slowly cooked such as on a spit, which allows germination of heat resistant spores and multiplication of vegetative cells, and trypsin inhibitors such as in sweet potatoes (a major part of the diet in Papua New Guinea) may result in infection.

3.5.5. Treatment

Apart from enteritis necroticans (section 3.5.4.), illness caused by *Cl. perfringens* is of short duration and is self-limiting. Recovery is usually complete within 24-48 hours and no treatment is required.

3.6. *Escherichia coli*

Escherichia coli is a part of the normal microflora of the intestinal tract of humans and most other warm-blooded animals so that it is generally present in faeces. Most strains of *E. coli* are harmless, but a few are pathogenic. They are Gram-negative, non-spore forming rods and are generally motile by peritrichous flagella, but there are some nonmotile strains. Many strains produce capsules.

The three principal antigens used for serotyping are the somatic antigen (O), the capsular antigen (K), and the flagellar antigen (H). To date, in excess of one hundred and seventy O antigens have been recognised although there may be others as yet unidentified. There are ninety known capsular antigens and fifty-six known flagellar antigens for serotyping *E. coli*.

There are principally four different groups of *E. coli* associated with food-borne disease:

- enteropathogenic (EPEC)
- enteroinvasive (EIEC)
- enterotoxigenic (ETEC)
- enterohaemorrhagic (EHEC/VTEC).

The first two are groups where the actual pathogenic mechanisms remain under investigation whereas ETEC and EHEC (VTEC) produce the symptoms related to illness via toxin production. VTEC is a so-called 'emerging' food-borne pathogen and will be discussed in more detail in Chapter 4.

3.6.1. Isolation and detection

Selective media for the isolation of *E. coli* make use of the ability of the organism to survive and multiply in bile. MacConkey agar is the traditional media for use in isolation although it is not extremely selective for *E. coli* and supports the growth of other organisms including some Gram-positives such as staphylococci. Eosin/methylene blue agar provides a more effective selective method of isolation and allows differentiation.

Immunologic tests have also been developed to determine the presence of *E. coli* toxins. These include enzyme immunoassays, radioimmunoassays, and other *in vitro* tests. PCR tests for the virulence factor genes also provide a means of identification in epidemiological studies.

3.6.2. Illness

The symptoms of illness caused by all four types of *E. coli* are shown in Table 3.2. Enteropathogenic *E. coli* (EPEC) is prominently known as a cause of outbreaks of neonatal diarrhoea. Many adults are asymptomatic carriers of EPEC and have developed immunity. Enteroinvasive *E. coli* (EIEC) infections have a similar pathology to those of *Shigella*. They also have some biochemical and serological similarities.

Table 3.2. Symptoms of illness caused by different types of *Escherichia coli*.

Type of pathogenic *E. coli*	Incubation time (average)	Duration of illness (average)	Symptoms
Enteropathogenic (EPEC)	17-72 hours (36 hours)	6 hours - 3 days (24 hours)	diarrhoea, nausea, vomiting, fever, chills
Enterotoxigenic (ETEC)	8-44 hours (26 hours)	3-19 days	profuse, watery diarrhoea, dehydration, vomiting, abdominal pain
Enteroinvasive (EIEC)	8-24 hours (11 hours)	days to weeks	fever, abdominal cramps, chills, profuse diarrhoea (sometimes bloody), headaches
Enterohaemorrhagic (EHEC)	3-9 days (4 days)	2-9 days	severe abdominal pain, vomiting, no fever, bloody diarrhoea, haemorrhagic colitis, haemolytic uraemic syndrome

The most common serotype of EPEC is O124 that has the same somatic antigen as *Shigella* O3. Because of this similarity, it may be that many cases of reported shigellosis may actually be due to enteroinvasive types of *E.coli*. Experiments with adult human volunteers have suggested that the infectious dose is quite high, generally 10^6-10^8 organisms. The ingested organisms invade the gut epithelial cells and multiply within them. Ulcerations of the colon result and hence bloody diarrhea.

Symptoms of enterotoxigenic *E. coli* (ETEC) are similar to those of cholera. The infectious dose may be quite high, between 10^8 and 10^{10} cells. This organism colonises the epithelial surface of the small intestine and produces one or more toxins that act on the small intestine resulting in an outpouring of fluid. ETEC does not invade or damage the epithelial layer of the small intestine. Certain requirements must be fulfilled for the ETEC to produce a diarrhoeal response in a host:

- the organism must contain the plasmid (a small piece of DNA that is 'extra' to the organism's primary DNA) that codes for one or two toxins
- the host must ingest a sufficient number of the organism to produce illness (probably about 10^6 or more)
- the organism must be in contact with the mucosa of the small intestine accomplished through colonisation factors.

ETEC can produce one of two types of toxin or both, depending on their plasmid content. One toxin is known to be heat labile and is inactivated in 30 minutes at 60°C. Heat-stable toxins, of which there are several types, able to withstand 100°C for 30 minutes are also expressed by some types of ETEC. Another important feature of ETEC is colonisation factors. These colonisation factors are very specific fimbriae that are filamentous appendages on the surface of the cell wall that allow the ETEC to adhere to the intestinal epithelial cells. A variety of types of species-specific colonisation factors have been identified. This means that an ETEC type which causes disease in animals cannot cause disease in humans and vice versa.

61

3.6.3. Epidemiology

Serotyping is an important feature of all epidemiological studies because it allows the source of contamination to be identified which is essential for control and future preventive measures. This is particularly true in the case of *E. coli* because of the potential seriousness of the illness caused. Fortunately food-poisoning by EPEC, EIEC and ETEC is relatively uncommon in the UK and USA. EPEC has mainly been associated with outbreaks in nurseries although a few food-related outbreaks of EPEC diarrhoea have occurred in adults. ETEC is generally more commonly associated with travellers' diarrhoea than it is with food-borne disease. The epidemiology of ETEC will be discussed in more detail in Chapter 4.

3.6.4. Vehicles of infection

Humans are the main reservoirs of the enteropathogenic, enteroinvasive, and enterotoxigenic types of *E. coli*. Infected individuals excrete the organism in their faeces, which ultimately contaminate food. The contamination generally occurs via contaminated water or from contact with infected food handlers. Serious problems with these three types of *E. coli* occur in developing countries, where unsanitary conditions exist and where untreated human sewage may contaminate water used for drinking or irrigation of food crops.

Enteropathogenic *E. coli* caused an outbreak in the United States in 1968 due to drinking of unchlorinated well water apparently contaminated by human sewage. Several food-associated outbreaks have occurred in England and Wales linked to eating cold, previously cooked meat and meat products. However, this organism is a rather infrequent cause of food-borne disease. EIEC may be spread by water and food and by person-to-person contact. Not many food-borne outbreaks have been linked to EIEC, but salmon, poultry, milk, and soft cheeses have been reported as vehicles.

Enterotoxigenic *E. coli* is the most common cause of "travellers' diarrhea" accounting for about 60-70% of all cases. There have been several food-borne outbreaks due to ETEC. These have been related either to an infected food handler or to use of water contaminated by sewage. ETEC may be transmitted via water, either by drinking, or even swimming in, water contaminated with raw sewage. Person-to-person contact may also be a means of transmission although there is only circumstantial evidence for this.

3.6.5. Treatment

Illnesses caused by these three types of *E.coli* are usually self-limiting and do not require antibiotic treatment.

3.7. Listeria monocytogenes

The numbers of reported cases of *Listeria*, particularly *Listeria monocytogenes*, in the UK have remained at a relatively low level since the peak that occurred in 1988-1989. The majority of cases are sporadic and often the source of contamination is unknown. Since *Listeria monocytogenes* was first described in 1926 other members of the genus have been identified including *L. innocua*, *L. welshimeri* and *L. seelegri*. However, only *L. monocytogenes* has been associated with pathogenesis. *L. monocytogenes* is a Gram-positive, non-sporing, facultatively anaerobic rod that can grow at temperatures between -0.4°C and 50°C. The organism is widespread throughout the environment being commonly found in water, soil, animals and vegetation and has been isolated from cattle, goats, poultry and sheep (although not usually from wild animals) and also from human and animal faecal waste.

3.7.1. Isolation and detection

Traditionally *L. monocytogenes* was isolated from environmental samples such as food using a cold-enrichment technique. However, because of the long incubation periods involved in this technique, selective media have been developed using a cocktail of antibiotics that, together with incubation at higher temperatures, results in a more rapid isolation for routine analysis of samples. Generally these selective media incorporate aesculin and ferric ammonium sulphate so that, because of its ability to hydrolyse aesculin, colonies of *L. monocytogenes* appear black or dark brown. Further biochemical tests such as sugar fermentation tests are necessary to confirm the colonies as *L. monocytogenes*.

Several ELISA and DNA probe methods are available commercially but these still require pre-enrichment although they are generally more rapid than the established confirmatory methods.

3.7.2. Illness

Listeriosis is an atypical food-borne disease with the gastrointestinal symptoms typically associated with food-borne pathogens not usually occurring. However, these symptoms may occur in mild cases in healthy individuals with similar doses causing more serious illnesses such as meningitis, meningoencephalitis or sepsis in those who are immuno-compromised.

Listeriosis cases are defined as either non-pregnancy-associated, which refers to all cases aged more than one month and unassociated with pregnancy, or pregnancy-associated. Adverse effects in pregnancy include spontaneous abortion, stillbirth or premature labour. Early (within first five days of life) or late (neonates aged 6-28 days) onset infection is often associated with a history of maternal influenza-type illness prior to delivery.

3.7.3. Epidemiology

The number of pregnancy-associated cases has declined to around 26% of all cases in 1996 compared with 31% in 1983 and 48% in 1989. The overall rate of listeriosis remained at between 1.6 and 2.7 per million population between 1983 and 1996 which means that the number of non-pregnancy-associated cases, especially in immunocompromised individuals, is increasing steadily. Cases associated with pregnancy fell to 0.1 to 0.2 per 10 000 conceptions in 1995 compared with 0.4 to 0.7 per 10 000 between 1983 and 1986.

Figure 3.1. Cases of pregnancy associated and non-pregnancy associated listeriosis in England and Wales 1983-1997 (compiled from CDSC data).

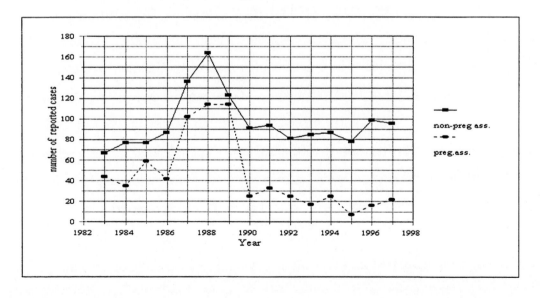

Listeriosis in humans occurs mainly sporadically but several epidemics have occurred. The incidence of *L. monocytogenes* infection in England and Wales is low (Table 3.1.) Nevertheless, the mortality rate is high (about 30% for non-pregnancy associated) and the adverse outcome rate in pregnancy-associated cases is approximately 30%. Between 1987 and 1989, the incidence rate increased by more than 200%. This increase was largely due to the contamination of pâté manufactured at one plant that was removed from point of sale. Once it had been identified, the number of cases decreased. Epidemiological studies of selected areas of the UK suggest that, compared with the reported incidence of other causes of food poisoning, the reported numbers of cases of listeriosis are probably an accurate reflection of the actual incidence rate.

3.7.4. Vehicles of infection

The most frequent transmission route for listeriosis is the consumption of contaminated food with the main sources of *Listeria* infection being fresh vegetables, prepared salads, raw poultry and soft cheeses, pâté and other cooked meat products and fish. There is also an epidemiological association established between consumption of either undercooked hot dogs or chicken and human listeriosis. Levels of contamination and incidence rates vary with type of food. In general fresh meats tend to contain <100 organisms g^{-1} with higher numbers being found in processed meat and poultry products. In a small survey in 1989 in the UK 6.7% of salad ingredients samples (ten out of 150) and 19% of mixed salad samples (eight out of 42) were found to be contaminated with *Listeria monocytogenes* with levels being <200 g^{-1}. Highest risk foods are often ready-to-eat, stored at refrigeration temperatures for long periods and contaminated with a high level of *L. monocytogenes* (>100 g^{-1} or ml^{-1}). Low levels of the organism may be initially present in an environmentally stressed condition but a long storage time may allow the organism to recover and multiply. The USA position is that of zero tolerance to the presence of the organism. In the UK, although this is an aim, the PHLS suggests that $<10^2$ g^{-1} may be considered fairly satisfactory (Table 3.3). Epidemiological studies have suggested that the human infective dose is between 10^6 g^{-1} and 10^9 g^{-1}, although for those that are immuno-suppressed such as cancer patients the infective dose may be lower.

Household refrigerators are used to store produce naturally contaminated by *Listeria* spp. and several studies have reported high frequencies and levels of contamination. Since *L. monocytogenes* is able to adhere to a variety of surfaces used in refrigerators such as glass it may be able to survive for long periods in a biofilm becoming a source of contamination within the domestic environment.

Table 3.3. PHLS guidelines for ready-to-eat food samples at a point of sale.

	L. monocytogenes detected in 25 g sample
Satisfactory (the aim)	Not detected
Fairly satisfactory	Present at $<10^2$ g^{-1}
Unsatisfactory	Present at 10^2 -10^3 g^{-1}
Potentially hazardous/unacceptable	Present at $> 10^3$ g^{-1}

Although thorough cooking kills *Listeria* spp., foods kept in the refrigerator and not subsequently cooked may provide a source of contamination especially under conditions of mild temperature abuse and long storage times. The prevalence of *L. monocytogenes* may not be high in foods such as ready-packaged salad and minimally processed vegetables, seafood and smoked fish products but it may be higher in dairy foods.

3.7.5. Treatment

Early detection of the presence of *L. monocytogenes* is necessary for successful treatment. The antibiotic erythromycin is often administered to pregnant women to reduce the presence of the bacterium, whereas penicillin or ampicillin plus gentamicin is generally the treatment of choice for otherwise healthy individuals.

3.8. Shigella

The *Shigella* genus consists of four species *Sh. dysenteriae*, *Sh. flexneri*, *Sh. boydii* and *Sh. sonnei* all of which are considered human pathogens. This genus was first described as the cause of bacillary dysentery in 1898 by Kiyoshi Shiga, a Japanese scientist. They all cause dysentery in humans although the severity of disease varies with *Sh. dysenteriae* being the cause of large outbreaks of severe dysentery in tropical countries whereas *Sh. sonnei* causes the mildest symptoms and is common in the USA and Europe where *Sh. dysenteriae* is rarely found. The other two species cause symptoms of intermediate severity.

3.8.1. Isolation and detection

Shigellae do not survive very well outside their natural habitat of the gastrointestinal tract of humans and other primates. They grow in a wide range of temperatures (10-45°C) and in a pH range of 6 to 8. The organism may be readily isolated from situations where human faecal contamination has occurred such as seepage of untreated sewage, or soiling. *Shigella* has not attracted as much interest as other food-borne pathogens with the result that laboratory isolation techniques have not been developed to such an extent as for *Salmonella* and others. Pre-enrichment procedures using selenite broth or Gram-negative broth have been suggested for isolation from food and clinical samples. Selective plating techniques using general Enterobacteriaceae or *Salmonella* media are generally used although neither produce satisfactory results. More specific isolation techniques developed include immunoassays for the virulence antigen and detection of specific genes using the polymerase chain reaction although, again, these are costly and time consuming.

3.8.2. Illness

Shigella causes illness via two pathogenic mechanisms:

- invasiveness
- enterotoxin production.

The organism is able to proliferate in the gut lumen, invade the gastrointestinal mucosa and multiply within the cells although it rarely causes bacteraemia. However, red blood cells may infiltrate into the lumen, resulting in characteristic bloody stools.

The enterotoxin (also called Shiga toxin) produced by some Shigellas such as *Sh. dysenteriae* serotype 1 has a range of biological activities. It has neurotoxic activity as well as being a very effective protein synthesis inhibitor. Since the toxin is proteinaceous, it is heat-labile and should be inactivated by adequate cooking. Shiga-like toxins or 'verotoxins', are produced by certain strains of *Escherichia coli*.

Shigella food-poisoning (or shigellosis) may vary in severity from asymptomatic infection to full-blown dysentery depending on the species of shigella involved. When the causative organism is *Sh. dysenteriae,* there is often abdominal pain, fever and the frequent passage of bloody/fluid stools and the patient may also have headaches, nausea and undergo prostration. Alternatively, if the organism responsible is *Sh. sonnei,* there may only be a mild diarrhoea without fever. The incubation period may vary from one to seven days, but is usually less than four days after ingestion of contaminated food.

3.8.3. Epidemiology

The majority of outbreaks of shigellosis worldwide are associated with drinking contaminated water but food-poisoning outbreaks caused by shigellae also occur and there have been some large outbreaks reported particularly in the USA. Since the organism is not a natural inhabitant of the environment, infection originates from individuals in the acute phase of illness as well as those who are asymptomatic such as those previously infected and recovering, or those who are excreters but remain healthy. *Sh. sonnei* is the most common cause of illness in the UK and also the least virulent. Other shigella such as *Sh. dysenteriae, Sh. flexneri* and *Sh. boydii* cause limited numbers of cases that are more serious in nature.

The low infective dose reported for *Shigella* spp. of 100 bacteria or less means that care in personal hygiene is very important in transmission of infection. A minor lapse in hygiene procedures may have serious consequences. In developing countries adequate chlorination of water supplies and the safe disposal of sewage would result in the numbers of cases of infection due to *Shigella* spp. decreasing substantially.

3.8.4. Vehicles of infection

Contact with human faeces transmits shigellae. Water may easily become contaminated due to inefficient drinking water treatment or the seepage of sewage through the earth. Raw fruit and vegetables may become infected by shigella if such contaminated water has washed them or by using soiled hands. In all cases where foods have been implicated in transmission, they will almost always have become contaminated by human faeces. A range of foods have been implicated both as the source of outbreaks and of sporadic cases including potato salad (a major vehicle in USA), shellfish, cheeses, rice and other vegetables and milk. One of the major risk factors for contamination of food vehicles is a large amount of handling before consumption, for example chopped, mixed, salads. Many studies have shown shigellae to be able to survive in foods at temperatures as low as -20°C for some time depending on the type of food involved. At refrigeration temperatures of 4°C the organism can survive in butter and margarine for up to 100 days and in eggs and milk for up to fifty days. In the UK secondary cases are not uncommon especially in kindergartens or creches and in 'poor housing, multi-child' households.

3.8.5. Treatment

Shigellosis is usually self-limiting and recovery often complete within one to two weeks after the onset of symptoms. However, those individuals from susceptible groups such as the very young, very old and/or debilitated patients with severe diarrhoea caused by *Sh. dysenteriae*, for example, may undergo serious, potentially fatal dehydration, which requires immediate treatment. If anti-microbial therapy is necessary then the antibiotic sensitivity of the causative organism should be determined before treatment is started because of the ability of the organism to become antibiotic resistant.

3.9. *Staphylococcus aureus*

Staphylococcus was first suspected in association with food-poisoning in 1884 but this was not confirmed until 1914 when it was demonstrated that human illness occurred by consuming stored, unrefrigerated milk from a cow with staphylococcal mastitis.

These bacteria are Gram-positive, facultatively anaerobic, non-spore-forming cocci that are able to grow over a range of 7°C to 48°C and produce an enterotoxin over a slightly narrower temperature range. The organism has a normal heat resistance and is able to grow between pHs of 4 and 10. However, it is unusual in that it is able to survive at low water activities as well as at high salt concentrations. Some strains have been reported as growing at 20% salt concentrations. The toxin itself is heat-stable and only inactivated by prolonged boiling. This means that care must be taken to reduce risk of growth (and therefore toxin production) in food cooked and consumed without further heat treatment.

3.9.1. Isolation and detection

Colony growth on Baird-Parker (B-P) agar gives a preliminary screening method for identification of *Staph. aureus* with characteristic jet black colonies surrounded by a clear zone. The two further confirmatory tests used to distinguish *Staph. aureus* from other staphylococci are the coagulase test (coagulase is an extracellular substance which coagulates human or animal blood in the absence of calcium) and the thermostable nuclease test (breakdown of DNA by a nuclease which has survived boiling). Two other coagulase positive *Staphylococcus* spp. are *Staph. intermedium* and *Staph. hyicus*. The former produces white colonies on B-P media (i.e. is unable to reduce the tellerite present) while the latter may only be differentiated from *Staph. aureus* by a series of biochemical tests.

Enzyme linked immunoassays and latex agglutination tests are used to identify staphylococcal enterotoxins and, although when initially developed these produced a high false positive rate, the latest commercially available tests are more reliable.

3.9.2. Illness

Food-poisoning caused by *Staph. aureus* is characterised by nausea, vomiting, abdominal pain and sometimes prostration. Diarrhoea is a common symptom but generally without fever occurring approximately one to six hours after ingestion of contaminated food. The symptoms are caused by the ingestion of food containing preformed enterotoxins secreted by the organism. Eight different types (A, B, C1, C2, C3, D, E and F) have so far been recognised. Although generally referred to as enterotoxins their actions are as neurotoxins. They stimulate the endings of the vagus nerve in the intestine and thus the vomiting centre in the brain.

The toxins are produced during multiplication of the organism in foods especially during inappropriate storage. Each toxin is relatively heat-stable and remains toxic after heating to 100°C for up to thiry minutes which would kill the organisms themselves. The enterotoxin most frequently involved in food-poisoning is staphylococcal enterotoxin A (SEA) which is found in the food associated with approximately 75% of outbreaks due to *Staph. aureus* with SED being the second most important cause of staphylococcal food poisoning outbreaks.

3.9.3. Epidemiology

Staph. aureus is a harmless parasite found on human body surfaces. However, it can cause minor skin complaints such as abscesses and, if the skin barrier is breached or host resistance particularly low, becomes an opportunistic pathogen. It is a common cause of food-poisoning in the USA but relatively uncommon in UK (Table 3.1.). The frequency of outbreaks may be linked to dietary habits so that those countries with widespread consumption of commercially prepared foods and/or a high frequency of large communal meals have an increased frequency of outbreaks. However, because *Staph. aureus* food-poisoning usually produces transient symptoms with rapid recovery, the reported numbers may not reflect the true incidence. In epidemiological studies the consequence of the high carriage rate (25-50% of the population may carry *Staph. aureus*) has sometimes made the identification of the source of an outbreak difficult. However, because the majority of the strains responsible for food poisoning belong to serogroup 111, the spread of infection can be more easily monitored than if they all belonged to different phage groups. Phage typing of the organism linked with enterotoxin identification are important epidemiological tools for tracing the source or sources of contamination in outbreaks.

3.9.4. Vehicles of infection

Staph. aureus is a major pathogen of man causing a wide range of infections, and can be found as a commensal on the skin and in the anterior nares of the nose. Coughing and sneezing of food handlers may result in contamination of food by this organism. *Staph. aureus* is usually transmitted to food from a human source or by cross-contamination from utensils, food preparation surfaces etc. previously contaminated by humans. The presence of small numbers of *Staph. aureus* on food is common. It occurs as a normal part of the microflora on poultry skin for example and as such may pose a risk of cross-contamination to other foods which are already cooked or will be consumed without further cooking. Contamination alone is not enough to cause an outbreak since more than 10^6 organisms per gram of food are typically required for infection but storage (particularly at ambient temperature) after contamination has occurred is an important risk factor in allowing enterotoxin to develop. Since the enterotoxin may not be subsequentially inactivated by the further heat treatment of the food, if any, this poses a risk to the consumer. Avoiding a delay between handling and cooking is not always possible and consumption but ensuring minimal handling and keeping foods refrigerated prior to cooking or serving will reduce significantly the risk to the consumer.

Foods commonly implicated in this type of food poisoning include cooked foods eaten cold such as processed meats and eggs, and prepared foods such as custards and other dairy produce. Foods with a high salt content, such as ham, have also been associated with *Staph. aureus* food-poisoning since the organism is able to grow in the levels of salt used in processing such foods particularly when competing flora are inhibited.

3.9.5. Treatment

Most patients infected recover completely within 24 hours without specific therapy. The mortality rate is low but in about 10% of cases the symptoms are serious enough for hospital admission to occur.

3.10. Vibrio

Vibrio cholerae is the type species of this genus. They are short, comma shaped, motile Gram-negative organisms that are facultative anaerobes. *V. cholerae* is able to grow in a temperature range of 15-42°C, ideally between 30 and 37°C. It grows between pH6 and pH10 but dies off rapidly in the presence of acid. It will grow in the presence of up to 6% sodium chloride but not higher concentrations, unlike other members of the genus.

V. cholerae strains belonging to two serogroups based on their ability to be agglutinated by a single antiserum O1 related to a somatic antigen. *V. cholerae* O1 are more often involved in the epidemics of cholera that occur in developing countries but O139, a more recently described serotype is also associated with cholera-like illness. The non-O1 strains are those that are non-agglutinable although some produce cholera toxin.

There are two other members of the genus associated with food-poisoning incidents. *V. parahaemolyticus* has the same cell morphology as *V. cholerae* but is an obligate halophile (i.e. it requires sodium chloride for growth) as is *V. vulnificus*, another member of the genus.

3.10.1. Isolation and detection

When numbers of vibrios are expected to be low such as in environmental samples, a pre-enrichment procedure is necessary for detection and enumeration. Alkaline peptone water (pH 8.5) is effective for these purposes. Plating out on selective media such as thiosulphate-citrate bile salts sucrose (TCBS) after incubation at 37°C for between six and eighteen hours results in an effective method for isolation of vibrios. Further identification can be made by morphology and biochemical tests such as oxidase (+) and sucrose fermentation. Commercial kits have been developed for rapid identification of vibrios although these are not completely reliable. *V. cholerae* serogroup O1 is subdivided into two biotypes, *V.cholerae* and *El Tor*, based on such properties as haemolysis of sheep red blood cells, agglutination of chicken red blood cells, polymyxin B sensitivity, and Group IV phage sensitivity. These biotypes are further serotyped based on some somatic antigen factors: Ogawa, Inaba and Hikojima. The other major group of *V. cholerae* are the non-O1 strains, which are sometimes called the nonagglutinating O:I *V. cholerae* (NAG) and sometimes the non-*Vibrio cholerae* (NVC).

Clinical isolates of *V. parahaemolyticus* may be serotyped for epidemiological purposes using a scheme based on 11 thermostable O (somatic) antigens and the 65 thermolabile K (capsular) antigens.

3.10.2. Illness

The disease caused by *V. cholerae* (O1 and O139) is cholera, characterised by profuse, watery diarrhoea sometimes described by physicians as "rice water stool." The symptoms also include abdominal pain and very rapid, severe dehydration, which results in intense thirst together with very cold and clammy skin. An individual at the height of illness may lose several litres of fluid in a day. The onset time for cholera is about two days. The infectious dose has been estimated at 10^8-10^9 cells although certain strains are more virulent than others. Ingestion of as few as 10^3 cells of some *El Tor* strains after the stomach acidity had been neutralised with bicarbonate has been known to produce illness.

This organism colonises the gut in a similar way to enterotoxigenic *Escherichia coli,* though the mechanism remains undetermined. The organism produces a toxin that causes an outpouring of fluid into the gut by a specific mechanism involving binding to a receptor on an enterocyte (cells lining the gut epithelium), a protein subunit entering the cell and changing the permeability of the cell membrane to various ions including sodium, potassium and chloride. A massive outflow of water into the lumen occurs, resulting in the classic profuse diarrhoea and subsequent dehydration of the host. Non-O strains produce a milder gastroenteritis which has as symptoms nausea, vomiting, abdominal pain and fever.

A watery diarrhoea is the most common syndrome produced by *V. parahaemolyticus* which has an incubation period of four to ninety-six hours (average fifteen hours) and a duration of three days. This organism may also produce a dysentery syndrome with mucus and blood in the stool. The incubation period maybe as short as two hours although nine to twenty-five hours is more usual with a normal duration of about two days. The infectious dose is usually high, requiring ingestion of more than 10^5 cells. Mechanisms of pathogenicity of *V. parahaemolyticus* are not well understood but most strains that are clinical isolates are positive for the so-called Kanagawa phenomenon. That is, these isolates produce a haemolysin that is able to lyse rabbit or human red blood cells but not horse blood cells when grown on "Wagatsuma agar," A thermostable hemolysin is responsible for the Kanagawa phenomenon. In contrast, most food isolates are Kanagawa phenomenon negative.

V. vulnificus is associated with three separate disease processes:

- an invasive process resulting in septicaemia with a mortality rate of about 50%. This is rare in normal healthy individuals with the majority of cases, if not all, being identified in individuals with an underlying previous illness such as liver disease and diabetes
- a tissue infectious process generally caused by infection of a wound from a contaminated aquatic source including during the cleaning of shellfish
- a gastrointestinal illness caused uniquely by consumption of raw oysters.

3.10.3. Epidemiology

Cholera is endemic in the Indian subcontinent where it is a major cause of death. Pandemics in the 19th century which spread from South-East Asia to Europe resulted in the development of a sewage and water treatment system which is the foundation of our system today. The present pandemic (the seventh) began in 1961 in Indonesia and has spread to Africa and reached South and Central America where nearly 400 000 cases were reported to WHO in 1991.

V. parahaemolyticus is responsible for a large percentage of cases of food-borne gastroenteritis in Japan probably related to the traditional Japanese diet although it is rare in the UK. *V. vulnificus* infection tends to be concentrated in countries whose sea-waters remain warm for most of the year although even in these geographical areas infections are very rare.

Vibrio parahaemolyticus has worldwide distribution; it is part of the normal flora of estuarine and coastal waters. It is believed to be primarily transmitted through seafood. It grows very rapidly in seafood that is temperature abused; for example, in raw squid at 30° C a generation time of fifteen minutes has been reported. It is sensitive to cold storage and dies off during refrigerated (4°C) or frozen (-10°C) storage.

3.10.4. Vehicles of infection

Vibrio cholerae is quite widely distributed in marine environments. There was a cholera outbreak in the USA in 1978, the first in the United States since 1911. Investigations revealed that the organism was in crabs that had been improperly cooked. More recently, there have been cases and outbreaks of cholera from eating raw oysters. *V. cholerae* O1 appears to be present in our marine environments, but to a lesser degree than are non-O: I strains.

The epidemic types of *V. cholerae* are thought to be mainly transmitted through humans. The organism is carried in the intestinal tract and excreted by symptomatic and some asymptomatic individuals and is present in their faeces, often at levels of 10^2-10^9 per gram. Faecal contamination of water or food results in transmission. Water is generally implicated more often than food as a vehicle of infection, but recent studies have shown that shellfish may also provide a reservoir of epidemic-type *V. cholerae*. The organism can survive in shellfish for long periods and has been isolated from moist portions of mussels, crabs and prawns.

Non-O strains are common contaminants of shellfish and most cases are associated with consumption of shellfish. This is a particular problem when the shellfish is from warm waters when the organism may be able to multiply to high levels. Both *V. parahaemolyticus* and *V. vulnificans* infections are also associated with consumption of shellfish.

3.10.5. Treatment

Without treatment cholera may be fatal especially in those individuals who are malnourished or immuno-compromised. The copious diarrhoea associated with infection by *V. cholerae* O1 and O139 rapidly results in severe dehydration, hypertension and salt imbalance. Recovery is dependent on the patient receiving rehydration therapy and is usually complete within six days. *V. vulnificans* infections require antibiotic treatment for effective recovery.

3.11. *Yersinia enterocolitica*

The genus *Yersinia* contains eleven species, the most important of which in terms of human infections is *Yersinia enterocolitica*. *Y. enterocolitica* is a Gram-negative facultative anaerobic rod-shaped organism. Although the optimum temperature for growth is 37°C, it is able to grow at temperatures of domestic refrigerators. It exhibits a number of phenotypic temperature-dependent characteristics. For example, it is nonmotile at 37°C but motile at temperatures below 30°C.

3.11.1. Isolation and detection

Various procedures have been developed for the isolation of *Y. enterocolitica*, the majority of which have depended on the ability of the organism to grow at low temperatures. However, as with *Listeria* spp., this resulted in a long incubation period with the attendant risk of overgrowth by other pyschotrophic organisms, which has not been found to be satisfactory for routine use.

Phosphate buffered saline or tryptone soya broth are often used for the pre-enrichment stage (4°C for twenty-one days) while for direct isolation from foods or from the pre-enrichment media CIN (cefsulodin/irgasan/novobiocin) agar or BOS (bile/oxalate/sorbose) have both been shown to give consistent results. The majority of isolates from food are nonpathogenic strains (otherwise known as environmental strains) and so further tests must be used to distinguish these strains from pathogenic *Y. enterocolitica*. These tests have included serotyping, biotyping and phage typing which are helpful in terms of identifying pathogenic strains since pathogenicity only appears to be related to certain types which are also specific to geographical areas. Development of gene probes to detect the virulence-associated plasmid for routine use may provide a specific method for detection of pathogenic *Y. enterocolitica* without the necessity for prolonged incubation times and enrichment methods, but as yet these techniques are not used routinely.

3.11.2. Illness

Gastrointestinal symptoms are most commonly experienced in food-poisoning caused by *Y. enterocolitica* and may include abdominal pain, fever and diarrhoea. The latter may persist for several weeks. Other reported symptoms include: bloody stools, nausea, headache, malaise and vomiting. The type and severity of the symptoms depend on the virulence of the strain involved and the immune status of the individual. Children of less than seven years of age seem to be the most vulnerable.

Acute joint pains due to acute inflammation of the connective tissue are reported in a minority of those infected and in a further minority of cases complications involving a chronic inflammatory response may occur such as ankylosing spondylitis and rheumatoid arthritis. In these latter cases, about one in one thousand of those initially infected, the organism cannot be isolated but antibodies can be detected.

The mechanism by which *Y. enterocolitica* causes symptoms involves, adhesion to the mucosal cells, invasion of the epithelial cells and phagocytes resulting in damage to the epithelial surface and malabsorption and hence diarrhoea. A heat-stable enterotoxin is produced by most clinical isolates but its contribution to the pathogenesis is undetermined.

3.11.3. Epidemiology

The prevalence of food-poisoning cases caused by *Y. enterocolitica* varies between countries. In the 1980s the organism was considered an 'emerging' food-associated pathogen because reported cases, mainly sporadic, in the UK increased by more than ten fold from 45 in 1980 to 590 in 1989. The figures for the 1990s do not show that it has become a major contributor to the figures for England and Wales. Cases are more common in colder climates such as northern Europe and, interestingly, show a different seasonal pattern from other food pathogens with a peak in reported cases occurring in autumn and winter.

3.11.4. Vehicles of infection

Pigs are the main environmental reservoirs of *Y. enterocolitica* and consumption of undercooked pork and pork products has been shown to be a major risk factor in developing yersiniosis. However, since most cases are sporadic, the sources of the infection have very rarely been identified. Care should be taken when handling parts of the pig carcass that may be contaminated with the organism. This includes pork chitterlings (pig intestines) which is a delicacy in certain communities. It has been recommended that these types of products should not be served to children less than seven years of age.

Y. enterocolitica is able to survive a wide range of adverse storage conditions such as freezing at -16°C to -17°C for six months in meat and refrigeration at 4°C for three weeks. The ability of the organism to survive and subsequently multiply at low storage temperatures depends on the nature of the food and the presence of competing microflora. At high salt or low pHs, growth of *Y. enterocolitica* is inhibited. At slightly abusive temperatures of 5°C to 8°C spoilage microflora outgrow *Y. enterocolitica* so that the food appears spoilt before the organism is able to multiply to pathogenic levels.

3.11.5. Treatment

In the majority of cases antibiotic treatment is not required because the illness is self-limiting. However, in severe cases prompt treatment is necessary to prevent further complications such as those already described developing.

CHAPTER 4

EMERGING BACTERIAL FOOD-BORNE PATHOGENS

4.1. Introduction

During the last decade a number of organisms have been either definitely identified as being, or are thought to be, food-borne pathogens. These are either new strains of already well-researched organisms such as *Escherichia coli* (*E. coli* O157) or newly identified organisms such as *Arcobacter* spp. They have been described as 'emerging' food-associated pathogens and although numbers of cases may be relatively small at the moment, as other organisms are effectively prevented from entering the human food chain, these 'emerging' pathogens provide the next challenge for the surveillance services and those involved in control and prevention.

4.2. *Escherichia coli* O157

The first report of *E. coli* O157: H7 as a human pathogen, which occurred after an outbreak of food-poisoning in the USA in 1982, was caused by individuals eating contaminated hamburgers from a fast-food restaurant. Since then it has become a major cause of diarrhoea, haemorrhagic colitis and haemolytic uraemic syndrome in many countries. In the UK numbers of reported cases have been increasing steadily during the last decade (Figure 4.1.) and world-wide it is becoming an important public health issue in terms of the number of outbreaks and associated high mortality rate.

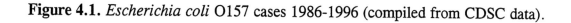

Figure 4.1. *Escherichia coli* O157 cases 1986-1996 (compiled from CDSC data).

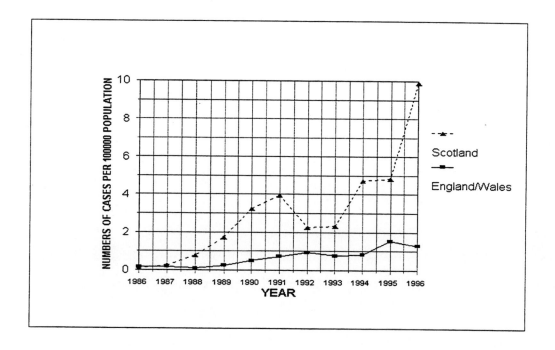

4.2.1. Symptoms of infection

E. coli O157 is a highly virulent organism which produces a toxin once established in the lining of the intestinal tract. Depending on the strain, either verocytotoxin type 1 (VT1) or verocytotoxin type 2 (VT2) is produced, or in some cases both. In 1996 75% of isolates in England and Wales were VT2 producing strains, 0.6% were VT1 and 23% were both VT1 and VT2 producing.

The symptoms caused by *E. coli* O157 vary from patient to patient. Young children, the immuno-compromised and the elderly are most susceptible to *E. coli* O157 infection. In mild cases the clinical symptoms consist of diarrhoea with some nausea, intense abdominal pain but little or no fever. Haemorrhagic colitis (HC) may develop and, in serious cases, haemolytic uraemic syndrome (HUS). Microangiopathic haemolytic anaemia (fragmented blood cells) and thrombocytopenia (low platelet count) are associated with HUS which is fatal in 3-5% of patients and has been identified as the main cause of kidney failure in children in the UK. About half of the patients infected with *E. coli* O157 do not have blood in the faeces and may develop HUS without previously showing symptoms of HC. In order to diagnose such patients as at risk from HUS it has been suggested that all diarrhoeal stools should be screened for *E. coli* VTEC.

4.2.2. Epidemiology of E.coli O157

E. coli O157 cases generally occur as family or general outbreaks. The largest series of outbreaks world-wide occurred in Japan in 1996 with approximately 10 000 people affected and a number of suspect foods identified, the main source of contamination being uncooked radish sprouts. In the case of an outbreak in the USA in 1993 which affected 732 individuals the food source was under-cooked hamburgers.

In the UK the largest outbreak was one that occurred in Scotland in 1996 when over 400 were infected resulting in nearly twenty deaths. Of the first 110 cases eighteen were children of which several had serious kidney damage. A study of this incident revealed some important features of how easily infections may be spread in a community. The first cases were noted in November 1996 and many of these and subsequent cases were in the same town. Health officials identified the probable source as cooked meat from a particular butcher who not only supplied his own retail premises but also a wide range of other retailers and wholesalers. This resulted in a potentially large population being at risk. The meat was purchased pre-cooked and the primary cases were those who consumed the *E. coli* infected meat. Secondary cases were also reported, for example, a nurse involved in the care of some of the affected patients and a policeman who investigated the outbreak as well as family members who did not consume the original contaminated cooked meat. This demonstrates the ease with which the organism is able to spread in a community unless very careful hygiene measures are established.

Within the UK there are regional differences in infection rates. Lower rates are generally reported in England and Wales compared with Scotland (Figure 4.1.) and also with other parts of the world especially regions of Canada. Investigations into the reasons for these differences may lead to a further understanding of the epidemiology of the organism and its environmental reservoirs.

4.2.3. Detection

The increasing number of reports of *E. coli* infections is partially due to improving methods of detection and surveillance. At the present time there is universal testing of all laboratory specimens. Detection of the organism in possibly contaminated foods is important for effective surveillance programmes especially considering the infective dose of *E. coli* O157 may be as low as ten cells. In foods, because of the probability of low numbers of *E. coli* O157 but large numbers of other organisms present, highly selective culturing procedures have been developed. In faeces of infected patients the numbers of the organism are usually high, making direct culture methods more appropriate. A number of detection regimes have been evaluated (Table 4.1.) with most recommending an enrichment procedure for isolation from both food and faeces to shorten detection time and minimize costs.

Typing of strains is important in epidemiological studies and a combination of phage typing and toxin gene typing combined with a range of DNA based techniques such as PCR may result in enhanced identification of sources of infection and monitoring of outbreaks.

Table 4.1. Some methods of isolation and detection used for *E. coli* O157

Type of sample	Method of detection
Faeces of dairy herds	pre-enrichment in modified tryptone-soya broth and culture on Chromagar[R]
Beef	immunomagnetic separation
Heat/freeze-stressed cells	selective plating using modified sorbitol McConkey agar, modified eosin methylene blue agar
Minced beef	Dynabeads[TM] enrichment: growth on CT-SMAC agar
Faeces of wild birds	pre-enrichment in modified tryptone-soya broth, growth on Chromagar[R]: confirmation on CT-SMAC agar

4.2.4. Reservoirs in the environment

The major source of *E. coli* O157 is cattle which are mainly infected early in life. Although these infected cattle are asymptomatic they shed the organism into the environment in faeces for some time. Contamination of the meat at the slaughter house from intestinal contents has been identified as a means of entry into the human food chain. This may occur from faeces on the hide or from spillage of the intestinal contents during preparation of the carcass. The risk of the former can be reduced by presenting 'clean' animals for slaughter and of the latter by bagging of the anus or oesophageal sealing. Possible cross contamination of carcases may be reduced by allowing adequate space on conveyer belts between each one and separating those with hides and those which have been skinned.

Beef is not the only source of *E. coli* O157. Contamination rates of 1.5-2% of other fresh meats on retail sale have been reported which may suggest that poultry, sheep and pigs may also harbour the organism. However, cross contamination from cattle at the abattoir or beef at the point of sale may also be a reason for these findings. Outbreaks have been associated with the consumption of raw milk and with post-processing contamination of pasteurised milk. Similar strains of VTEC have been found in a number of human cases and in contact farm animals showing an association between infection in children and their previous recreational visit to farms where they handled cattle and goats.

Although cattle are the main environmental reservoir with transmission from animal to animal or animal to human a major means of infection, the distribution of *E. coli* O157 in the environment as a whole is relatively unknown and other transmission modes remain to be determined. *E.coli* O157 has been isolated from faecal samples of a small percentage of gulls at an urban landfill site and from intertidal sediments (0.9% and 2.9% respectively) in Northern Britain but whether this reflects a direct route into the human food chain or merely an indirect one via cattle remains to be investigated.

The majority of cases especially in the USA have been caused by eating beefburgers. This is probably related to the processing involved in their production (i.e. mincing, mixing etc.) which increases the distribution of the organism, if present, to a larger number of food products and hence to a wider consumer population.

4.2.5 Control and prevention

Although control of VTEC illness in humans requires identification of contaminated carcasses at the slaughterhouse which is not a feasible option, entry of uncontaminated meat into the food chain would result in a reduction in *E. coli* infections in the population. A number of end process treatments have been investigated for reducing numbers of *E. coli* O157 on beef carcasses with differing degrees of effectiveness (Table 4.2.). Moist heat interventions such as hot water washes and application of steam-vacuum have been shown to add a degree of safety to beef products when *E. coli* spp. are present on the carcass surface at high levels. Proper heat treatment of raw milk and adequate cooking of raw meat and other foods will ensure safe products since the organism is killed by heating to an internal temperature of 68.3°C. *E. coli* O157 is probably not able to grow at refrigeration temperatures of below 5°C but this depends on the initial inoculum, the food product and the time of storage.

Table 4.2. Examples of post-slaughter decontamination regimes.

Treatment	Effectiveness
Chlorine (NaOCl) spray	reduction of < 1 log (10) at 50,100, 250, 500 ppm; 1.04 log (10) at 800 ppm
Trisodium phosphate	reduction of 3 log (10)
1% fumaric acid at 55°C, 5s.	reduction of 1.3 log (10).
Hot water/steam	reduction of 3.4 log(10)

In the case of *E. coli* O157 the low infective dose means that personal and food hygiene procedures must be robust in order to reduce, if not eliminate, the risk of cross contamination from infected raw food to that which will be consumed without further cooking. The Pennington report recommended that in retail premises raw and cooked food should be separated at all times including, if possible, the use of separate staff.

4.2.6. Conclusion

E. coli O157 is a cause of serious illness in humans. An overall HACCP approach at the farm, slaughter-house, during processing and retail sale will result in the risk of *E. coli* O157 infection being substantially reduced. Thorough cooking of raw meats, correct pasteurisation of raw milk and avoidance of risky procedures in terms of cross-contamination will provide effective means of preventing infection.

4.3. *Arcobacter* spp.

The *Arcobacter* genus was suggested in 1991 for bacteria which had been previously classified as aerotolerant *Campylobacters*. The rRNA Superfamily VI of bacteria contains three closely related organisms: *Campylobacter, Arcobacter* and *Helicobacter* (see section 4.4.). *Arcobacter* is differentiated from the other two members by its ability to grow at 15°C and its aerotolerance.

Arcobacter was first isolated from bovine aborted foetuses and has been subsequentially isolated from aborted porcine foetuses and cows with bovine mastitis. At the present time two species have been associated with human illness: *Arcobacter cryaerophilus* and *Arcobacter butzleri* with the latter being the most frequently reported. The clinical significance and epidemiology of these organisms are unknown at present.

4.3.1. Symptoms of infection

The symptoms of illness caused by *Arcobacter* are similar to those of *Campylobacter* infection. They include abdominal pain (with or without diarrhoea), nausea and fever. *A. butzleri* has been isolated from patients with enteric symptoms with no underlying disease and from those with enteritis **with** underlying disease so that there seems to be no association with immune system dysfunction.

4.3.2. Epidemiology of Arcobacter

Since clinical specimens are not routinely examined for *Arcobacters,* very little is known about the epidemiology of the organism. It may be that a large number of undetermined cases are actually those caused by *Arcobacters* but the prevalence remains to be established. The fact that *Arcobacters* require a lower isolation temperature than *Campylobacters* has probably meant that lack of appropriate culture techniques has resulted in under-reporting of the prevalence of this organism. Transmission may involve:

- drinking contaminated water associated with travel
- consumption of contaminated food
- person-to-person contact,

but the major mechanisms are undetermined at present.

4.3.3. Detection

Isolation of *Arcobacter* spp. from animal tissues has proved difficult. Although, unlike *Campylobacter*, *Arcobacter* does not require microaerophilic conditions for growth, primary isolation from environmental samples such as food is more efficient if low oxygen concentrations (3 to 10%) are maintained. Secondary passage may be achieved in aerobic conditions.

Use of blood based media is necessary for isolation although these are not selective for *Arcobacter* so that the organism may be overgrown by other bacterial flora present in the sample. Several non-blood based media have been assessed for reliability of isolation from environmental samples. Modified cefsulodin-irgasan-novobiocin (CIN) agar and others such as CAT and CCDA (section 2.2.1), with modifications especially for *Arcobacters*, are being developed and evaluated for routine use. Incubation at 37°C (*Arcobacter*) or 42°C (*Campylobacter*) allows differential use of these media.

4.3.4. Reservoirs in the environment

Arcobacter is relatively widespread in the environment although, to date, infection has mainly been associated with consumption of pork and pork products. It has been isolated from a wide range of animal sources including live animals and meat including chickens and beef.

A. butzleri has been detected in drinking water reservoirs in eastern Germany and from canal waters in Thailand. Its presence in unchlorinated water supplies suggest that this may be a major means of transmission. Other studies involving small outbreaks of the illness caused by *A. butzleri* suggest a person-to-person route of transmission.

4.3.5. Control and prevention

As in the case of most pathogenic bacteria, proper cooking procedures kill the organism so that the risk to human health **may** be negligible, although cross-contamination to already cooked foods and those foods which are consumed without cooking may still provide a risk to human health.

4.4. *Helicobacter pylori*

This organism was first described and named in 1983 although the presence of curved bacilli in the gastric epithelium had been observed for many years. *Helicobacter pylori* is a Gram-negative, spiral, microaerophilic rod and is the only known organism that is able to survive and multiply in the human stomach. It does this by adhering to the gastric epithelium and generating a micro-environment in which it is able to survive. The micro-environment is achieved by the production of urea which neutralises the acid of the stomach in that particular part of the stomach thus allowing growth of *H. pylori*.

4.4.1. *Symptoms of infection*

H. pylori associated gastritis is now known as the most common chronic infectious disease in the world, affecting about 50% of the population. Many individuals infected with the organism are asymptomatic and never develop disease. However, *H. pylori* is associated with 90% of cases of duodenal ulcers although its role in the development of peptic ulcers is less well established. *H. pylori* infection is a risk factor in the development of gastric cancer. Infection, once established, persists for many years and even life, if not treated effectively. Progression to gastric cancer is obviously dependant on co-factors such as genetic predisposition, smoking habit, alcohol consumption or diet.

4.4.2. *Epidemiology of infection by H. pylori*

H. pylori has been detected in nearly every population in the world either by direct isolation or by indirect measurements such as antibody titres or urea breath tests. Prevalence of infection varies with various factors:

- age (older age groups have a greater prevalence)

- gender (more females are infected than males, all other factors being similar)

- populations in developing countries have higher prevalence

- in developed countries it is associated with specific race or ethnic groups

- over-crowding (particularly in childhood)

- socio-economic factors in general (lower socio-economic grouping the greater prevalence).

In the UK and USA the prevalence at age 20 is 20% but at 55-60 years of age 50% of the population are infected. In developing countries, on the other hand, 50% are infected by the age of 20.

4.4.3. Detection

Infection by *H. pylori* is detected by various methods:

- endoscopy and subsequent biopsy of gastric mucosa

- direct culture

- detection of anti-*H. pylori* antibodies

- urea breath test.

The latter is dependent on the fact that infection by *H. pylori* results in the production of large amounts of urea in the stomach. This may be detected by a breath test. The only difficulty with this is that it produces a high false positive rate so that if symptoms persist one of the other methods of detection should be used.

H. pylori is difficult to grow in the laboratory routinely since it is a fragile organism which does not survive easily outside its human host. The use of blood based media (e.g. tryptone-soya agar supplemented with horse serum) as well as microaerophilic conditions and a long incubation period results in the most effective isolation regime.

4.4.4. Reservoirs in the environment

Humans were thought to be the only natural host of *H. pylori*. However, recently it has been isolated from non-human primates and from cats. This suggests that it may also be a zoonotic pathogen with a possible transmission route from animals to humans. However, epidemiological studies have not linked exposure to animals with *H. pylori* infection in humans. Person-to person spread is the most likely means of transmission although the organism has been detected in drinking water and vegetables. Its presence has been detected in dental plaque and in faeces suggesting a oral-faecal route of transmission. The likelihood of *H. pylori* being a food-borne pathogen remains although its main transmission route is unknown and person-to person spread is the most reasonable assumption. However, it may be because isolation and detection methods are not well developed or sensitive enough that the organism has not been shown to be a food-borne pathogen at the present time. The potential remains for *H. pylori* to be characterised as a food-borne pathogen in the future.

A proportion of household flies have recently been found to carry some of the *H. pylori* genome suggesting that insects may be an primary source of infection in humans, or at the least, involved in the cross-contamination of food.

4.4.5. Control and prevention

Treatment with a cocktail of antibiotics results in eradiation of the organism from the stomach. This results in healing of, for example, gastric ulcers, and hence relief of symptoms. The most commonly prescribed regimes are those including amoxycillin and metronidazole or clarithromycin. Since the actual mechanisms of spread are unknown, preventative measures are difficult to institute. Eradication is therefore the one effective means of control.

4.5. Conclusion

This chapter has concentrated on the 'emerging' (or potentially 'emerging') food-borne pathogens. As more pathogens are eliminated from the human food chain others might emerge. This might be because previously they were out-grown by the major food-poisoning organisms or because the now established organism mutates in order to survive. With the adaptability of bacteria it seems that humans will always have to deal with risks from pathogenic bacteria and their transmission into the human food chain.

CHAPTER 5

FOOD PRESERVATION TECHNIQUES

5.1. Introduction

The best method of arresting the increasing rise in food poisoning cases is a concerted attack at all stages of food production and processing from 'farm to fork'. The ideal situation would be that pathogenic micro-organisms are completely eradicated from food but, because of the ubiquitous nature of many micro-organisms of concern, this is probably unachievable and could not be sustained throughout the food chain. Although an increase in food quality may not reduce the numbers of **reported** cases, it would probably have an effect on the underlying burden on the community in terms of unreported illness and days' work lost.

Consumer demand for food, particularly fresh produce, with a long shelf-life has corresponded to a dramatic change in food purchasing habits. Weekly (or less frequent) trips to the supermarket have almost totally replaced the corner shop and the daily purchase of fresh foods, common until the1970s. Consumers expect a wide choice of foods at the supermarket including convenience foods and are more discriminating than previously. While recognising the safety issues, the discerning shopper also requires food that is more 'natural' or less heavily processed and preserved. This provides the food industry as a whole with a problem: how do you ensure food safety without extensive processing and the use of chemical preservatives?

Substantial advances have been made in understanding the effects of various preservation techniques on both food spoilage micro-organisms and food pathogens. The application of HACCP programmes to food processing has improved the overall quality of food in terms of safety. This chapter examines both traditional and novel preservation and packaging techniques and considers their effect on the bacterial flora present in the food.

5.2. Why preserve food?

Ever since our ancestors discovered that they could prolong their supply of meat and fish by drying it in the sun, humans have been attempting to preserve food to reduce the differences between supply and demand, especially at certain seasons. Smoking, pickling and salting have given way to newer methods such as chilling and freezing. However, consumers' requirements are continuously changing and the food industry has responded with new packaging and preservation techniques, designed to provide both variety and quality, whatever the season.

In terms of microbiological stability foods may be divided into three types:
- stable - those that do not spoil microbiologically because they do not contain water that is necessary for growth, e.g. chocolate, flour, sugar
- semi-perishable - foods that when stored in correct conditions such as low temperatures without initial damage will keep for some time, e.g. potatoes, apples
- perishable - those foods that even at low temperatures will spoil in short periods due to the microbial flora initially present on them, e.g. strawberries and other soft fruit.

For both consumers and the food industry the features of a 'good' preservation technique would include:

- long shelf-life

- no change in organoleptic properties of food

- use of fewer chemicals

- use of less packaging

- wide range of foods available.

Table 5.1. Objectives of different food preservation techniques.

Objective	Technique
Inhibition or slowing down of growth	Chilling
	Freezing
	Drying
	Modified atmosphere packaging
	Addition of chemical preservatives
	Sous-vide cooking
	Pickling
	Vacuum packaging
Inactivation	Canning
	Irradiation
	Addition of bacteriocins

Early preservation techniques included the use of chemicals, chilling/freezing, canning, dehydration or combinations of these. For various reasons these techniques have given way to novel methods of food preserving and packaging such as modified atmosphere packaging, irradiation, sous-vide packaging and the use of bacteriocins.

Apart from preventing access of micro-organisms to the food product in the first instance, there are two main precepts of food preservation techniques. One involves the inhibition or slowing down of the multiplication of food spoilage microbial flora and also, hopefully, the proliferation of any pathogens present. This is achieved by changing the conditions that favour microbial growth. The other relies on total inactivation of the microbial flora present in the food (Table 5.1.).

5.3. Brief review of 'traditional' technologies

This section provides a brief overview of the preservation techniques used more traditionally within the food industry.

5.3.1. Chemical preservatives

A preservative is defined as: **a substance that is capable of inhibiting, arresting or retarding the process of fermentation, acidification or other deterioration of food or the masking of evidence of putrefaction of food.** The mechanisms by which preservatives carry out this process may be:

- by producing a barrier between the food and the environment
- by providing an environment in which micro-organisms are unable to survive and multiply
- by interfering with the biochemical processes of the microbial flora present on the food.

Table 5.2. Some preservatives used in food.

Preservative	Action	Active against	Example of use in foods
Acetic acid	Reduces pH	Bacteria, moulds, yeasts	Pickles, sauces
Benzoic acid	Reduces pH	Moulds, yeasts	Soft drinks, cider, fruit products
Sorbic acid	Reduces pH	Moulds, yeasts, catalase-positive bacteria	Salad dressing
Nitrite	Interferes with metabolism particularly energy producing mechanisms	Bacteria (used especially to inhibit *Clostridium botulinum* and other spore forming bacteria which survive heat treatment)	Cured meat and meat products
Sulfur dioxide	Disrupts DNA, RNA and proteins so affecting metabolism	Gram-negative bacteria, moulds, yeasts	Fresh sausage meat

Although the addition of chemicals, whether natural or artificial, to food is regarded by a proportion of the public as a perversion of all that may be considered 'natural', the use of many preservatives is a well-established part of Western culture. For example, smoked fish and meat are relatively common dietary constituents. Levels of preservatives added to food are more carefully controlled by law nowadays then ever before and their usage is in overall decline. However, this control produces its own problems since at the low concentrations allowable in food most preservatives only slow rather than totally inhibit growth of micro-organisms. Thus preservatives tend only to be really useful when initial contamination of the food is low. Good hygiene practices remain essential during all stages of subsequent processing.

5.3.2. *Canning*

This is probably the most important food preservation technique worldwide, both in terms of tonnage produced and also the variety of foods for which it is used. Changes occur in food processed by canning. Nutrients such as vitamins are lost and there are also changes in organoleptic properties. Some foods, for example, soft fruits, do not maintain their original taste and texture.

The main problem organism in the canning industry is the anaerobic pathogen *Cl. botulinum*. If this organism (or its spores) are present in the food before canning the resultant canned food provides favourable conditions for *Cl. botulinum* survival and multiplication. Another problem for the canning industry, and one which has been a common source of human infection in the past, is that of post-processing contamination. This may occur after heat-treatment as a result of the water used to cool the can being forced through insufficient seals into the food by negative pressure. The canning process consists of heating food with a temperature/time combination to allow the destruction of the *Cl. botulinum* and its spores. This technique, known as **commercial sterilisation**, is in comparison to true sterilisation which would mean heating the food at a temperature/time combination to allow the destruction of **all** known organisms and their spores. Certain thermophilic spore-forming micro-organisms produce heat resistant spores. Nevertheless, these organisms do not multiply below 45°C and so do not pose a risk at normal storage temperatures. The food industry has invested a large amount of resources into producing a relatively trouble-free canning process which results in safe food and, since the 1970s, there have been very few outbreaks of food-borne disease due to consumption of food canned in the UK.

5.3.3. Dehydration

This method of preservation relies on the fact that micro-organisms require water for growth so that reducing the water content will reduce or eliminate growth (but not necessarily survival). Properties of the food change so that this method is not suitable for all types of food. Dehydration techniques are used mainly for vegetables and vegetable-based products such as soups and sauces.

5.3.4. Chilling or freezing

All micro-organisms have a range of temperatures in which they are able to grow and multiply. This is different for each organism and some food-borne pathogens, such as *L. monocytogenes*, are able to grow at refrigeration temperatures while others, such as *E. coli* O157, can survive (but not multiply) at freezing temperatures of -20°C. Thus a reduction of temperature may be used to inhibit partially (chilling) or fully (freezing) growth of microbial flora. Freezing particularly changes the organoleptic properties of some foods, especially those with a high water content, such as soft fruits. However, there is little nutrient loss and chilled and frozen foods can be regarded as 'fresh' in terms of nutritional content.

'Quick freezing', where the thermal centre of the food passes through 0-4°C in thirty minutes, is the most efficient freezing method and is used in commercial circumstances. Home freezing, in which food can take seven to eight hours to reach 0°C at the centre, allows a greater survival of any microbial flora present.

5.3.5. Freeze-drying

This process involves drying of food under a vacuum. It is a relatively expensive process although it does have several advantages:

*   it can be used on heat sensitive foods
*   on rehydration the food resembles the food before processing
*   there are no nutrient losses
*   no discolourisation of the food occurs.

5.4. New techniques of food processing and packaging

There are several novel methods of food processing which have been developed in the last decade or so. The following sections describe the most common in use in the UK.

5.4.1. Modified atmosphere packaging (MAP)

The growth of aerobic microbial food spoilage flora and chemical oxidation reactions within the food are the two main reasons that food undergoes spoilage. Although chilling alone does reduce both the chemical effect of atmospheric oxygen and the growth of aerobic food spoilage micro-organisms, it does not increase shelf-life significantly. However, modifying the atmosphere surrounding the food in order to reduce oxygen changes the growth characteristics of the microbial flora present and results in an increased shelf-life. Techniques used to reduce oxygen around the food are known by the overall term **Modified Atmosphere Packaging (MAP)** and include vacuum packaging and controlled atmosphere packaging (Table 5.3.).

The first description of the effect of modified atmosphere packaging (MAP) was in 1927, when it was reported as increasing the storage life of fruit. MAP techniques have now been shown to increase the shelf-life of a wide range of products (Table 5.4.). However, it was not until modification techniques were introduced commercially in Europe in the 1970s, that there was a sharp increase in availability of MAP food products.

Table 5.3. Terminologies used in MAP (from: Phillips, 1996; reproduced with permission from Blackwell Science Ltd.)

Terminology	
Modified Atmosphere Packaging (MAP)	Replacement of air with a single gas or combination of gases. No further control over initial gas composition.
Controlled Atmosphere Packaging (CAP) or Controlled Atmosphere Storage (CAS)	Replacement of air with single gas or combination of gases with proportion and type of gas mixture controlled over the total storage time.
Equilibrium Modified Atmosphere Packaging (EMA)	Pack is flushed with gas or sealed without modification. Permeability of packaging and respiration of produce results in an equilibrium between the inside and outside of pack. Used mainly for fresh fruit and vegetables.
Vacuum Packaging (VP)	Product sealed in low gas permeability film after total evacuation of pack. Results in changes of atmosphere inside the pack during storage due to altered metabolism of product and microbial flora and gas permeation.
Vacuum Skin Packaging	Used for delicate products. Softened film placed over product and vacuum applied.

Table 5.4. Percentage increase in shelf-lives of foods using MAP techniques.

Food product	% increase in shelf-life for MAP over air stored, refridgerated products
Pork	100
Chicken	200
Beef	200
Fish	500
Cooked meat	300

Most packs for MAP products are made from one of more of four polymers: polyvinyl chloride (PVC), polyethylene terephthalate (PET), polyethylene (PE) and polypropylene (PP). There are various factors which must be taken into account when a film is chosen for a particular product:

- barrier properties and therefore permeability to various gases
- antifogging properties to allow good product visibility
- capacity to resist adverse handling such as resistance to tearing
- sealing ability both to itself and to the container
- special properties related to a product and its storage such as easy-peal seals for convenient opening or possibility of heating the product without removing it from packaging.

The permeability of the film used will determine whether the composition of the atmosphere inside the pack changes over storage time. If it is fully permeable then the atmosphere inside the pack will become the same as the air outside; if the film is semi-permeable, an equilibrium modified atmosphere results. Some films provide a barrier to movement of gases in both directions. If these are used for packaging fruit and vegetables, which continue to respire after harvesting and may contain high loading of microbial flora, anaerobic conditions may result. This situation is undesirable both because of the risk from *Cl. botulinum*, commonly present on vegetables, and because the product then changes organoleptic properties so that texture may change, i.e. it may shrivel. There have been suggestions that all MAP products should contain a low level of oxygen (5-10%) in order to decrease the possibility of growth of pathogenic anaerobic bacteria, particularly *Cl. botulinum*, but unless the packaging material is impervious to oxygen some oxygen will diffuse into the package during storage.

Models have been developed to allow the quantification of the consequences of the variability of pack properties such as number of micro-perforations per pack and the cross-sectional area of the perforations on gas concentration. These allow minimum homogeneity requirements for modified atmosphere packaging to be defined so that the effectiveness of new materials developed for MAP may be predicted.

Although the main gases used are oxygen, carbon dioxide and nitrogen (Table 5.5.), the type and proportion vary from food product to food product (Table 5.6.). The major factor in the anti-bacterial nature of MAP is the concentration of carbon dioxide present. Its effectiveness is influenced by the original and final concentrations of the gas, the temperature of storage and the original population of organisms. Microbial growth is reduced at high concentrations of carbon dioxide in a variety of products and this effect increases as storage temperature decreases. The anti-microbial activity of carbon dioxide is probably the result of the gas being absorbed onto the surface of the food forming carbonic acid, subsequent ionisation of the carbonic acid and a reduction in pH.

Table 5.5. The effects of gases used in MAP techniques.

Gas	Advantage	Disadvantage
Oxygen	Inhibits growth of anaerobes, e.g. *Cl. botulinum*. Keeps myoglobin in meat in oxygenated form giving the characteristic colour to red meat.	Stimulates growth of aerobic microbial flora which tend to be the main reason for food spoilage. Stimulates chemical oxidation processes causing rancidity.
Nitrogen	Inhibits growth of aerobic micro-organisms. Prevents pack collapse. Inhibits oxidative processes in food and thus rancidity.	
Carbon dioxide	Inhibits microbial growth. Effectiveness increases with decrease in temperature.	Dissolves in meat tissue resulting in pack collapse. High levels result in anaerobic conditions which may allow growth of *Cl. botulinum*, if present.

Other gases which have been suggested for use in MAP include nitrous and nitric oxides, carbon monoxide, sulphur dioxide, ethene and chlorine. However, most of these have not been developed for reasons which include safety, consumer response, legal aspects and cost.

Table 5.6. Some examples of atmospheres used in MAP products (from: Phillips, 1996: reproduced with permission from Blackwell Science Ltd).

Product	Atmospheres used
Bacon	20-35% CO_2: 65-80% N_2
Bakery products	100% N_2 /100% CO_2 20-70% CO_2: 20-80% N_2
Cheese	0-70% CO_2: 100-30% N_2
Cured meat	20-50% CO_2: 50-80% N_2
Fish (white)	40% CO_2: 30% O_2 : 30% N_2
Fish (fatty)	40-60% CO_2 : 40-60% N_2
Fruit/vegetables	3-8% CO_2: 2-5% O_2: 87-95% N_2
Meat (fresh)	30% CO_2:30% O_2: 40% N_2 15-40% CO_2: 60-85% O_2
Pasta (fresh)	100% N_2
Pasta (with meat)	50-80% CO_2: 20-50% N_2
Poultry (cooked)	30% CO_2: 70% N_2
Poultry (fresh)	100% CO_2 25-30% CO_2: 70-75% N_2 20-40% CO_2: 60-80% O_2 60-75% CO_2: 5-10% O_2: 20% N_2

5.4.1.1. Effects of MAP on overall product quality

The 'fresh' appearance of MAP-packaged food is maintained over relatively long periods because changes in sensory and colour characteristics, which are mainly caused by oxidative reactions, are reduced.

Raw fish particularly benefits from being packaged under modified atmospheres because MAP reduces production of chemicals such as peroxides. Since these chemicals affect the sensory characteristics, the shelf life of the product is increased considerably. However, **high** levels of carbon dioxide in packaging of fishery products may result in the carbon dioxide dissolving into the fish flesh causing deformation or collapse of the packaging. It also interferes with pigments in the flesh which affect the colour of the product.

Fresh fruits and vegetables are metabolically active for long periods after harvesting due to both intrinsic factors, such as respiration and other metabolic enzymic processes, and external factors such as physical injury, microbial flora, water loss and storage temperature. If the produce is sealed in impermeable film with low initial oxygen concentrations, anaerobic conditions may fairly quickly be established because the respiring fruit or vegetable uses the little oxygen that is present. When the oxygen is depleted to very low levels, anaerobic respiration of the fruit will be initiated which results in the accumulation of ethanol, acetaldehyde and organic acids and deterioration in organoleptic properties of the product. Each fruit or vegetable product requires a different gas combination as too little oxygen or too much carbon dioxide results in irregular ripening, browning or changes in organoleptic characteristics.

The maintenance of quality of a food product packaged in a modified atmosphere during extended times of storage is not only due to an inhibition of chemical reactions but also the growth of food spoilage micro-organisms. Gram-negative bacteria are generally more sensitive to high concentrations of carbon dioxide than are Gram-positive bacteria resulting in the inhibition of *Pseudomonas* spp. and the *Enterobacteriaceae* and domination of the gram positive lactic acid bacteria. The activity of these bacteria result in increased accumulation of acetate and lactate, decreased pH and enhanced tissue decay.

For the food producer and food manufacturer the shelf life of the product is a major consideration in terms of overall quality of the product. Modified atmosphere packaging will extend the shelf-life of many food products including ground pork, chicken carcasses, fresh and smoked fish, but not all, for example mushrooms or cooked, sliced ham.

5.4.1.2. *Effects of MAP on pathogenic bacteria*

Two factors may act to increase the risk from pathogens in MAP products:

- increasing the shelf-life of the product may allow environmentally stressed pathogens to recover
- inhibition of spoilage microflora may remove competition for the pathogens.

The safety of MAP food products in terms of pathogenic micro-organisms depends on whether the food is sold as 'ready-to-eat', requires minimal further heating or is raw. The use of MAP for any raw produce which is subsequently cooked is considered less hazardous because correct cooking procedures kill all pathogens.

Some bacteria (e.g. *Campylobacter* spp.), are not able to multiply on the food and in this case, as in all food processing procedures, it is essential to ensure initial contamination is kept to an absolute minium. Pathogens of particular concern are either those that are able to multiply at the refrigeration storage temperatures used for MAP products (e.g. *L. monocytogenes*) or those that are able to grow in anaerobic (or nearly anaerobic) conditions (e.g. *Cl. botulinum*). The food industry involved in producing MAP products has invested a considerable amount of money ensuring that the conditions used for each product decreases (if not eliminates) the possibility of contamination by such pathogens.

Growth of *L. monocytogenes* is inhibited in high levels of carbon dioxide at domestic refrigerator temperatures in a variety of products whereas growth of the anaerobe *Cl. botulinum* is favoured by MAP. Botulin toxin production can occur in atmospheres of up to 10% oxygen. The relationship between toxin production and organoleptic spoilage is important because if recognisable spoilage occurs before the food becomes toxic then there is no risk to the consumer. One recent study showed that when vacuum packaged raw beef was inoculated with spores of *Cl. botulinum* and stored at 25°C it was toxic at six days but by this time the meat had already spoiled and the consumer would not have attempted to eat it. Several studies have indicated that the overall incidence of the spores of *Cl. botulinum* in commercially available precut ready-to-eat MAP vegetables, at least, is low (0.36%) indicating that the possible anaerobic environment of MAP may not pose a potential health risk to the consumer in terms of *Cl. botulinum* toxin.

Salmonella spp. and *Campylobacter* spp. are both potential contaminants of food traditionally packaged by MAP such as poultry and dairy products. *C. jejuni* and *C. coli*, because they are microaerophilic, may be able to survive the low oxygen conditions of MAP. *C. jejuni* is not able to grow in carbon dioxide enriched atmospheres but may be able to survive. Thus, its presence in foods not subsequently cooked may present a hazard to humans. Modified atmospheres, combined with low storage temperatures, have been shown to have a bacteriostatic and bactericidal effect on *S. enteritidis* which suggests that it is probably not the introduction of MAP food products that has contributed to the increase in reported cases of food-borne salmonellosis in the UK and USA.

5.4.1.3. Recent developments in MAP

The most significant recent development in MAP technology is the development of 'intelligent' packaging systems to improve food safety. These systems may be defined as: **'integral components or properties of the packaging system which confer intelligence appropriate to function and use of the product itself and have the ability to sense or to be sensed and to communicate.'**

In most smart packaging chemicals are incorporated into the packaging (but not in contact with the food itself). These interact with the atmosphere of the packaging, the product characteristics or both, thus ensuring the optimum conditions are maintained and enhancing the shelf-life of the product. As a result of the interaction of the chemical and the atmosphere or product there is often a visible change in the characteristics of the chemical, usually of colour, which allows the consumer to monitor the safety and shelf-life of the food product so that they are able to assess the 'freshness' of the food. The use of oxygen scavengers together with oxygen indicators are an example of smart packaging techniques. Oxygen scavengers are easily oxidisable substances, such as powdered ferrous compounds or metallic platinum. These are contained in air-permeable sachets and incorporated into the packaging. When sealed with oxygen-impermeable films these generate an oxygen depleted atmosphere. If the pack also has an oxygen indicator included, the consumer will be able to assess the oxygen status of the packaging. An example of an oxygen indicator is the 'Ageless-eye[R]' a pill manufactured by the Mitsubishi Gas Chemical Company Inc. which is based on a chemical indicator reaction. When the atmosphere is low in oxygen (0.1% or less) the pill is pink and when the oxygen concentration higher (0.5% or more) the pill is blue allowing the consumer to judge at a glance the effectiveness of the packaging.

Ethyne is a gas formed by fruit and vegetables during storage and its presence encourages the ripening process. Reduction of ethyne within the packaging would increase the shelf-life of such fresh food considerably. Ethyne scavenger systems involve the use of potassium permanganate or activated carbon contained in sachets in the packaging. They remove the gas as it is formed thus increasing shelf-life of the produce.

The concentration of carbon dioxide in MAP fruit and vegetables can be kept within an acceptable range by the use of mineral salts which **absorb** carbon dioxide as it is formed by respiring fruit and vegetables. By changing the mineral salts used this system can be used to **generate** carbon dioxide in those circumstances where it is essential that carbon dioxide concentration is maintained within a set range but where it may be depleted by the necessary use of a semi-permeable film or by the generation of the gas by the product.

The inclusion of oxygen scavengers into food packaging has been opposed by some consumer groups because of the possibility of accidental consumption. There is also a basic mistrust of the use of 'unnecessary' additives in food products even if they do not come into contact with the food itself.

5.4.1.4. Conclusion

Although MAP has become a major packaging method for many foods, for example, 90-95% of fresh pasta sold in the UK is packaged using modified atmospheres, it does not increase significantly the shelf life of every type of food. Foods which undergo processing procedures such as smoking, already have long shelf-lives because of these prepackaging techniques. However, in these cases, use of MAP may improve other aspects of the food such as better colour stability or easier slice separation. Refrigeration is also required for most food products for MAP to be effective and safe. MAP does not enhance food quality. It is designed to inhibit the growth of whatever micro-flora are already present on the food at packaging. The combination of MAP techniques together with prior decontamination procedures such as the use of trisodium phosphate or gamma irradiation (Section 5.4.2.) may result in food which is both microbiologically safe and has a long shelf life. MAP techniques do not eliminate the necessity for proper, safe manufacturing procedures nor the need for careful handling at all stages from factory to table.

Concerns over safety, competition from high quality fresh food and vacuum-skin packaged food products and a prejudice against what might be regarded as 'excess' or unnecessary use of plastic packaging material have all meant that the expansion of MAP food in the marketplace has not occurred as might have been predicted in the 1980s.

5.4.2. Irradiation

As from 1st January 1991, consumers have had the choice of a new preservation technique which probably has not increased its market share as was expected. Irradiated food has been used for some time in specialised situations such as in hospital intensive care units and in space travel.

Table 5.7. Levels of radiation doses used in the irradiation of food.

Dose	Application
Low - less than 1 kilogray	To kill insects in cereals and fruit To control ripening To inhibit sprouting, e.g. potatoes
Medium - 1 to 10 kilogray	To reduce spoilage micro-organisms in food
High - more than 10 kilogray	To reduce bacterial contamination in general

The food industry advocates its use to prevent ripening of fruit and vegetables and also to eliminate pathogens from food such as poultry, which are known generally to have high contamination rates. It increases the shelf-life of soft fruit such as strawberries and inhibits the sprouting of root vegetables such as potatoes.

The technique uses a radiation source to irradiate the food. This is usually gamma rays from caesium-137 or cobalt-60. The source does not come into contact with the food at any stage of the procedure. There are three levels of radiation use depending on the application (Table 5.7.).

There has been controversy concerning the widespread use of irradiation techniques. However, there are a number of advantages to its use as well as disadvantages (Table 5.8.) which are relative to the type of food under consideration.

Table 5.8. Advantages and disadvantages of irradiation techniques.

Advantages	Disadvantages
Controls food-borne parasites	Does not kill viruses
Kills food-borne pathogens	Does not inactivate toxins
Loss of nutrients is minimal	Covers up bad hygiene practices
Increases shelf-life of food product	Does not inactivate enzymes which cause spoilage
Reduces need for use of chemical preservatives	Free radicals generated by irradiation cause oxidation of fats in food and may encourage rancidity
Ensures good quality product	Mutations may occur

5.4.2.1. Irradiation as an alternative to fumigation

Fumigation of food and food ingredients with various chemicals such as ethylene dibromide and ethylene oxide had been used for many years, particularly for controlling insect infestations. However, treatment of food with most of the previously used chemicals is now banned. This is for occupational safety, environmental or health reasons. For example, methyl bromide, used widely as a fumigant against insects and nematodes, has now been shown to be an ozone-depleting compound and so to add to worldwide environmental problems. Ethylene oxide is still allowed in some countries although its use is gradually decreasing. For those countries which rely on fresh food and food ingredients (e.g. dried herbs and spices) alternatives must be found in order for their economies to survive.

119

The combination of the ban of ethylene oxide by the EU in 1991 and the introduction of irradiated food laws in the UK, also in 1991, has meant that for certain foods, particularly spices, herbs and food seasonings, irradiation provides an effective means of ensuring food safety at a fairly reasonable cost compared with other treatments.

5.4.2.2. Irradiation as a method to ensure food safety

All of the food-poisoning bacteria mentioned in previous chapters are susceptible to irradiation at one to ten kilogray. Thus, it was argued by a WHO committee in 1986 that, considering that no other technique effectively controlled pathogenic contamination of some epidemiological important products such as poultry, the use of irradiation was the one means of ensuring safe food entered the human food chain. However, some pressure groups have suggested that its use might cover up bad hygiene practices which might become normal for food handlers involved, even when food is not going to be subsequently irradiated.

5.4.2.3. Irradiation as an energy saving process

Irradiation techniques compare well with other preservation techniques in terms of energy requirements. It is estimated that irradiation and subsequent refrigeration only uses one third of the energy required for keeping the food at freezing temperatures for the same time. After the year 2000 CFC refrigerants, used widely in the food industry, will not be available. This will result in increases in cost of cold (rather than chilled) storage making the differential between the two techniques even more.

5.4.2.4. Irradiation as a cost-effective process

Irradiation provides a cost-effective method for reducing the incidence of food-borne disease which itself is a burden on most countries in terms of healthcare expenditure, loss of working days and related costs. It also reduces microbial spoilage, premature ripening and physiological changes in food and thus post-harvest losses, which developing countries can ill-afford. Use of irradiation techniques facilitates the world trade in various commodities which, because of their perishable nature, would be confined to a more localised distribution. Insect infestation and food-borne parasites (which are outside the scope of this book) and post-harvest losses are controlled by low doses of one kilogray. Non-sporing pathogenic bacteria are killed by one to three kilogray generally without causing significant changes in organoleptic properties of the food. Therefore, although it may be a slightly more expensive process measured against other food preservation methods, when measured in terms of the world economy irradiation may provide a cost-effective preservation process overall.

5.4.2.5. Conclusion

Two major factors that have ensured that the widespread use of irradiation techniques has not occurred since its legalisation. First, although it is a relatively inexpensive technique in terms of running costs, it has high initial capital costs. Secondly, consumers have been extremely wary about buying products associated with irradiation because of adverse publicity.

However, because of the controversy and, in many countries, the active participation of all parties including consumers in the debate, irradiation has probably undergone the most scrutiny in terms of research and development of **all** food preservation techniques. Although its use has

121

not become universal, it has become established as a safe and effective method of food processing and preservation.

5.4.3. Sous-vide processing

This method of food processing is defined as: **raw materials, or raw materials with intermediate foods, that are cooked under controlled conditions of temperature and time inside heat-stable vacuumised pouches.** It is an example of the development of so-called cook-chill procedures where the food is cooked (usually as a recipe dish) and immediately cooled and a chill temperature (4-8°C) maintained until consumption. Overall lower temperatures and longer cooking times are used than in 'normal' cooking.

The major concern is that the conditions are not rigorous enough to eliminate heat resistant spores such as those from *Cl. botulinum* and so temperature control at all points of storage and a strict HACCP approach to production are essential to ensure food safety. The Advisory Committee on the Microbiological Safety of Food recommends:

- heat treatment at 90°C for ten minutes or equivalent at the core of the food
- a pH of 5 or less throughout product
- an a_w of 0.95 or less throughout the product
- a combination of processes that can be demonstrated to eliminate *Clostridium botulinum*, its spores and toxins.

There is some doubt over whether refrigeration alone is sufficient to guarantee the safety of sous-vide products. To address this issue the US Food and Drug Administration have recommended that:

- sous-vide products should have time-temperature recorders incorporated into their packaging to monitor the temperature history of the product

- in addition to the primary barrier of refrigeration, multiple barriers or hurdles should be incorporated into the sous-vide product.

Table 5.9. The advantages and disadvantages of sous-vide cooking.

Advantages	Disadvantages
More economic	Anaerobic conditions may result in growth of anaerobic pathogens such as *Cl. botulinum*
Nutrients are preserved	Heat resistant spores may not be killed
Reduces need for chemical preservatives	Application of HACCP approach at all stages of process including subsequent chilling absolutely necessary
Food has long shelf life	Pathogens allowed to recover from heat stress and multiply under long storage times
Little change in organoleptic properties of food occurs	

The extra hurdles would provide a combination of several factors which together ensure the safety of the food even though, taken alone, each of these would probably be insufficient to do so. Examples of such hurdles would be low pH, incorporation of organic acids, low water activity a_w and the use of protective cultures (see next section). Obviously the use of various hurdles depends on the food involved and there is much ongoing research in this area by food manufacturers to ensure sous-vide food safety.

5.4.3.1. Effect of sous-vide processing on pathogenic bacteria

Most of the research into the safety of sous-vide products has concentrated on the effect on spores of *Cl. botulinum*. Addition of sodium lactate to products containing beef, chicken or salmon as their their main constituents increased the time for toxin production. At pH 5.5 the addition of salt also inhibits toxin production for up to forty-two days of storage at 15°C. Generally the more 'hurdles' incorporated into the sous-vide product the lower the risk of microbial growth and therefore, for *Cl. botulinum*, the less risk of toxin contamination.

L. monocytogenes is another organism whose growth might be encouraged by the storage temperature of sous-vide food products. Irradiation at three kilogray combined with sous-vide cooking effectively eliminates the organism in that the pathogen has been shown to remain undetected in inoculated food samples after storage of eight weeks at 2°C. In uninoculated samples the use of irradiation on sous-vide products increases shelf-life from six to eight weeks. Therefore, the use of sodium lactate and/or irradiation in sous-vide products may ensure their safety.

5.4.3.2. Effect of sous-vide processing on spoilage microflora

Minimally processed food such as sous-vide products may originally contain high numbers of microflora which become thermally injured during processing. Under conditions of temperature abuse these may recover and be able to multiply to high numbers producing spoilage. Initially spoilage organisms are *Bacillus* spp. but after seven to ten days at 15°C the lactic acid bacteria become predominant resulting in an increase in carbon dioxide and lactic acid and a consequent decrease in pH. Thus swelling of the packaging and changes in organoleptic properties of the food may all be used to assess spoilage.

5.4.3.3. Effect of sous-vide processing on food quality

There are few published studies on the effects of sous-vide processing on sensory and nutritional aspects of food. Generally it is accepted that sous-vide cooking allows retention of vitamins and other nutrients, certainly compared with conventional methods of cooking such as boiling. Acceptability, in terms of sensory characteristics, is also higher, especially in vegetables such as broccoli. More research is required to determine which products benefit from sous-vide cooking as compared with traditional cooking and the conditions necessary to keep nutrient losses to a minimum.

5.4.3.4. Conclusion

In many countries sous-vide cooking is gaining in consumer popularity. It provides fresh-like products with potentially long shelf-lives together with the convenience of minimal cooking in the home. More research is required to clarify various aspects of the effects of sous-vide cooking and to determine factors such as additional hurdles to incorporate into the product and the ability of heat-stressed bacteria to recover during prolonged storage to ensure food safety. Other considerations in an extended research programme should be the determination of standard combinations of processing features such as pasteurisation values, cooling rates, storage times and temperatures and shelf lives and their effects on nutritional and organoleptic properties of sous-vide products.

5.4.4. Use of antagonistic bacteria and bacteriocins

Some recent research has indicated that antagonistic micro-organisms or their anti-microbial metabolites may have a role in the preservation of food. The latter are known as **bacteriocins** and may inhibit or kill the contaminants and thus prevent spoilage or the growth of pathogenic organisms. Bacteriocins are extracellularly released peptides or proteins that are bactericidal (or bacteriostatic) to bacteria closely related to the producer micro-organism. Biological preservation as an idea also includes the use of competitive microflora to reduce the growth of spoilage or pathogenic organisms in the food product plus the use of anti-microbial enzymes. Several possible strategies may be applied for the use of bacteriocins in food:

*   inoculation of the food with a starter or protective culture of lactic acid bacteria
*   addition of the purified or semi-purified bacteriocin as a food preservative
*   use of a product previously fermented with a bacteriocin-producing strain as an ingredient in food processing.

5.4.4.1. Bacteriocins produced by lactic acid bacteria

Lactic acid bacteria have been long associated with food fermentation and are generally regarded as 'safe'. They are able to exert a 'biopreservative' effect against other micro-organisms because of competition for nutrients and/or the production of bacteriocins and other antagonistic compounds such as organic acids and hydrogen peroxide.

Unfortunately bacteriocins from lactic acid bacteria are not active against Gram-negative bacteria such as *Salmonella* spp. although if their membrane is disrupted these organisms tend to be more susceptible. However, this is not generally practicable in food products.

126

Bacteriocins from a number of lactic acid bacteria are active against *L. monocytogenes* (Table 5.10).

Table 5.10. Bacteriocins produced by lactic acid bacteria active against *L. monocytogenes*

Product	Organism producing bacteriocin
Meat products:	
Salami	*Lactobacillus plantarum*
cured pork	*Lactobacillus sake* Lb 706
frankfurters	*Pediococcus acidilactici*
Dairy products:	
Italian cheese	*Enterococcus faecium*
Cheddar cheese	*Lactococcus lactis* subspecies *cremoris*
Vegetable-type foods:	
ready-to-use mixed salads	*Lactobacillus casei*
	Pediococcus (2 strains)

5.4.4.2. Foods used for bacteriocin-inhibited preservation

The majority of studies published to date relate to bacteriocins produced by antagonistic bacteria in meat and meat products particularly relating to *L. monocytogenes* inhibition. Problems arise in the use of bacteriocins in food since they first have to be approved as food additives. This can cause a particular problem with consumers because of the attitude to the addition of organisms to food.

Nisin is the only bacteriocin whose use has found industrial application on a large scale. It can be used instead of nitrate in foods and is commonly used in cheese spreads. Bacteriocin-producing lactic acid bacteria may be used in foods of plant origin, particularly mixed salad vegetables, especially as these products may have a high initial loading of microbial flora.

5.4.4.3. Conclusion

The use of bacteriocins or antagonistic micro-organisms in food products has had limited success to date. This is because many bacteriocins are less effective in foods than they are *in vitro*. Consumer ambivalence towards the addition of what may be considered extraneous micro-organisms to food products has compounded this. Also each bacteriocin must be characterised and accepted as a food additive in its own right making progress relatively slow. Food manufacturers have to be absolutely certain about the effect of the addition of such micro-organisms to food before serving them up wholesale to the consumer. The inhibitory mechanisms involved are relatively unknown and more research is required before widespread use of such a method is accepted as providing safe food within the human food chain.

5.5. Food preservation - the future

Food preservation techniques are expanding rapidly and it is important that legislation keeps pace with innovations. Novel methods must be thoroughly tried and tested before widespread use is initiated. It is obviously essential that food preservation techniques are in use to ensure high quality, safe foods at minimal cost to the consumer. However, the safety of food entering the human food chain is of primary importance and so extensive research must be initiated over any new methods that may be suggested by the food industry.

Although care at harvest and at slaughter limits microbial contamination of the food before any subsequent processing and packaging this is rarely an effective means of overall control in terms of safety. Primary contamination does occur and many foods contain the main organisms of concern such as *Salmonella* spp., *Campylobacter* spp., *L. monocytogenes* and *E. coli* O157. This will remain the situation for the foreseeable future. Food processors must therefore assume that these organisms are present in raw foods, perhaps not routinely, but certainly occasionally, and to consider this possibility in designing their procedures and packaging technologies. Any new (or even well established) methods of preservation must be shown to be effective in either inactivation or inhibition of the growth of the organisms of concern.

CHAPTER 6

FOOD SAFETY AND THE LAW

6.1. Introduction

As has been discussed in previous chapters it is obvious that bacterial food poisoning has become a major worldwide public health problem. The application of sound microbiological principles associated with proper safe practices at all stages of the food production process is the only method of ensuring the provision of safe food for consumers. This will result in the ultimate goal which is a reduction in the numbers of food-poisoning cases. In the UK there is a history of a number of pieces of legislation relating to a variety of aspects of food and its sale. These include laws designed to protect the consumer from: short measures (The Weights and Measures Act, 1985); defective products, including food products (The Consumer Protection Act, 1987); risk of illness or disease from animal sources (The Animal Health Act, 1981); spread of food poisoning (Public Health (Control of Disease) Act, 1984). With the increase in food-poisoning cases in the 1980s these measures were obviously not providing the basis for control.

6.2. History behind recent food safety law

In the late 1980s in the UK two food-poisoning bacteria attracted much media interest, and food safety in general became a public concern. *'Salmonella* in eggs' and *'Listeria* in soft cheese' were recognised by both public health authorities and the general population as serious health problems that should be addressed. Recently, in the 1990s, the so-called 'emerging' food-borne pathogens such as *E. coli* O157 have become everyday terms familiar to most of the general public. The ongoing debate concerning the epidemic of Bovine Spongiform Encephalopathy (BSE) in cattle and its possible implications for human health, which is outside the scope of this book, has also focussed attention on food safety issues.

Increased public awareness culminated in the recognition by government, and those involved in public health, for the need for more stringent controls and new legislation to enforce them. In 1989 the UK government announced the setting up of the Committee on the Microbiological Safety of Food, chaired by Sir Mark Richmond. The Committee was given the following broad terms of reference: **'To advise the Secretary of State for Health, the Minister of Agriculture, Fisheries and Food and the Secretaries of State for Scotland and Northern Ireland on matters remitted to it by Ministers relating to the microbiological safety of food and on such matters as it considers necessary.'**

The results of the deliberation of this committee, The Richmond Report, addressed specific questions relating to the increasing incidence of food poisoning in the UK, and attempted to establish whether this was linked to changes in agriculture, food production, food technology, retailing, catering and food handling in the home and make recommendations where pertinent. These recommendations were published in two parts: Part 1 in 1990 and Part 2 in 1991.

Part I covered public health matters including the incidence of food poisoning, human and food surveillance and outbreak management, as well as **poultry** meat production and manufacturing processes. The Richmond Report Part 1 recommended:

- further research on the natural history of listeriosis and the factors influencing the growth of *Listeria* spp. in different foods in order to determine preventative measures

- more studies aimed at finding the 'true' incidence of gastrointestinal illness, the related microbial cause(s) and possible food source(s)

- closer liaison between the Communicable Disease Surveillance Centre (CDSC) with data on human cases and the State Veterinary Service (SVS) which provides data on animal diseases in order to identify links between contaminated animal foods and the same pathogens causing human disease

- appointment of Consultants in Communicable Disease Control (CCDCs) by every District Health Authority to take overall responsibility for outbreak management

- further training of all relevant staff in the practical management of local and national outbreaks and all aspects of food safety

- more coordinated food surveillance studies at centres throughout the country, to provide national data on the microbiological quality of food

- common microbiological monitoring programmes to investigate the level of contamination at each stage in poultry-meat production

- further training of staff involved with food production, including the seeking of expert advice on food processes, which should be designed on HACCP principles

- the initiation of a registration or a licensing procedure that will include the inspection and approval of new premises for the production and/or sale of food

- the replacement of the present 'sell-by' labelling system of food by a uniform 'use-by' system.

Part 2 of the Richmond Report included an overview of the causes of food poisoning, identifying changes responsible for its increased incidence. Consideration was given to the microbiological hazards associated with **red** meat, milk, cheese and shellfish. The main recommendations included:

- the need to work towards a common definition of food poisoning not only for all countries of the UK but for the whole of the European Community

- an appeal for harmonisation of reporting of food poisoning statistics across the UK, whilst recognising the public health arrangements in Scotland and Northern Ireland;

- training of meat inspectors, Environmental Health Officers and veterinarians

- in the dairy industry, advice on the care required in cheese making with respect to listeriosis, following the implication of the consumption of unpasteurised milk as a major hazard

- an urgent need to look at the contamination of shellfish beds

- the setting up of a Code of Practice based on existing guidelines for all transport of refrigerated foodstuffs, to include vehicle monitoring facilities and adequate training of staff handling refrigerated foods

- the undertaking of new initiatives to review all microbiological safety aspects of retailing and wholesaling

- the maintenance of high standards in the planning and operating practices in catering, with special attention being given to HACCP guidelines

- the provision of advice to consumers on the optimal use of domestic refrigerators and microwave ovens

- the setting up of major new initiatives for improved education and training in food hygiene and food safety issues, related research to be encouraged nationally and with international collaboration.

Implementation of these recommendations was expected to make a significant impact on the level of microbiological contamination of food at all stages from 'farm to fork'. The legislation subsequentially put forward was based on the Richmond Report's main conclusions.

6.3. The Food Safety Act (1990) and Food Hygiene (Amendment) Regulations (1990)

The Food Safety Act 1990 that came into effect on 1st January 1991 was strengthened further by the Food Hygiene (Amendment) Regulations 1990 to allow legislative control of food and all premises involved in its production and consumption. There are heavy penalties for those that do not reach the prescribed standard (Table 6.1.) indicating the seriousness with which food safety offences are now regarded at government level.

Table 6.1. Penalties for offences under the Food Safety Act 1990.

Offence	Maximum penalty
Obstructing an enforcing officer, failure to give assistance or information	£2000 fine or three months' imprisonment or both
Rendering food harmful to health	£2000 fine or six months' imprisonment or both
Selling food that does not comply with safety regulations	£20 000 fine or six months' imprisonment or both
Selling food that is not of the nature, substance or quality demanded by the purchaser	£20 000 fine or six months' imprisonment or both
Other offences	A fine or six months' imprisonment or both

Except for the one dealing with obstruction, these penalties apply on summary conviction. For conviction on indictment, the maximum penalty in all cases is a fine or two years' imprisonment or both.

Local authority enforcement officers (both Environmental Health Officers and Trading Standards Officers) have been given several new powers under this legislation that have greatly enhanced their ability to deal with contraventions of the law quickly and efficiently. The Act provides for a wide range of regulations to be made in respect of many activities relating to food itself and also to food sources (animals, growing crops) and contact materials (packaging, containers) so that the interests of the consumer are protected and promoted. Twenty codes of practice have been issued under the Food Safety Act giving guidance to food authorities on the execution and enforcement of the Act and regulations and Orders made in relation to it.

The Food Safety Act (1990) and the Food Hygiene (Amendment) Regulations (1990) have provided a number of new concepts in food legislation.

6.3.1. Food safety requirements

These two laws define a new offence of selling, offering for sale, possessing or advertising for sale food that does not comply with a food safety requirement. Food fails a safety requirement if it is considered to be either harmful to health, or unfit for human consumption, or contaminated with materials that make it unfit for human consumption. If this is the case then the whole batch of food is presumed to be affected until the contrary is proven. The person responsible for the food (usually the owner of the business) is now liable for prosecution if he or she fails to ensure that it satisfies food safety requirements. Proper documentation of the 'lifetime' of the foodstuff including storage, processing and distribution is therefore required.

135

6.3.2. Food safety notices

Enforcement officers have been given very detailed and powerful new authorities for dealing with premises that contravene the legislation or pose a threat to the health of the consumer. At the time of inspection a notice may be served on the person committing the offence which may either give the recipient time to correct the fault (improvement notice) or may close down immediately the suspected (or proven) equipment, process or premises (prohibition notice). Since not to comply with a notice is an offence in itself, those individuals with the responsibility for a food business should be prepared to react quickly and positively on receipt of a notice and to limit the possibility of such a notice being served.

6.3.3. Registration of premises

Local authorities require all food businesses to register with them, and that not to do so is an offence. Licensing was a possible option favoured by many experts in the food safety field but the government considered this dictatorial and too costly to administer.

6.3.4. Food hygiene training

Hygiene training for every food handler is a necessity and certificated training at the level of the Institute of Environmental Health Officers Basic Food Hygiene Certificate or equivalent was originally suggested as a requirement. However, this obviously put a burden, both financial and otherwise, on food businesses so that it has become a requirement that each person involved in handling food is 'trained to the level required for the satisfactory carrying out of their occupation'. This allows individual food businesses to identify their own training needs and provide the necessary instruction depending on the type of operation and the job description of each employee. Some form of induction training together with regular updating and/or refresher courses is an absolute minimum.

Table 6.2. Rules for food handlers.

DO	DO NOT
Wash hands:	Smoke
after going to the toilet;	Chew anything
on entering a food room;	(including gum, tobacco,
after handling raw food;	fingernails)
after eating, smoking, coughing	Taste food being prepared
or sneezing;	Spit, cough or sneeze over food
after combing your hair;	Pick nose or ears
after handling waste or	Wear jewellery
chemicals.	Wear protective clothing outside
Keep fingernails short and	designated areas
clean.	
Cover cuts with waterproof	
dressing.	
Keep hair clean and covered.	
Wear clean protective clothing.	

Every food-handler should have an understanding of the basic principles of hygiene, why achieving it in practice is necessary and how this is accomplished. Such a course should include the following:

- micro-organisms as sources of food-spoilage and food-poisoning
- symptoms of infection by common food-poisoning organisms

- preventative measures for microbial growth, survival and contamination

- standards of personal hygiene (Table 6.2.)

- importance of proper handling and storage of foods including temperature regulation and measures to reduce cross-contamination

- effective cleaning procedures

- method for exclusion and control of common pests found in food premises

- outline of food safety laws.

6.3.5. Temperature regulation

The Food Hygiene (Amendment) Regulations (1990) provide the legislation for ensuring proper temperature control regimes are applied during receipt of food, storage, processing and distribution. Hot food has to be kept above 63°C and cold food below 5°C although this requirement is diluted by exemptions for certain categories of food, detailed in the DoH guidelines on the regulations.

6.3.6. The due diligence defence

'Due diligence' is a defence which may be claimed by those prosecuted under the Food Safety Act (1990) by local authority Environmental Health Officers. The 'due diligence' defence says 'it should be a defence for a person charged to prove that he or she took all reasonable precautions and exercised all due diligence to avoid the commission of the offence by himself or by a person under his control'. This allows the possibility of acquittal even when the facts show that an offence has been committed. However, in practice, in order to demonstrate to EHOs that such a defence exists, there must be a well-documented system for the provision, storage and handling of the food. This must be able to stand up to the strictest and most critical scrutiny. An example of such a system that **may** provide a defence is one that leads to accreditation by the British Standards Institute as a Quality Management System that complies with BS5750. The achievement of BS5750 will not automatically provide a defence, but it will give an indication to the court that the business is serious in its attempt to assure safety.

6.4. The James Report

Because of the increasing public debate concerning food and food safety issues, the then Leader of the Opposition asked Professor Philip James to make recommendations on the structure and function of a proposed new body to be known as the Food Standards Agency. The James Report was published in 1997 and recommended the following:

- the agency should advise Ministers on all matters relating to food safety, food standards, and nutrition and public health; its remit should encompass the complete food chain

- it should be a statutory Non-Departmental Public Body with executive powers, reporting to Parliament through Health Ministers, with the Secretary for Health taking the lead

- the agency should be governed by a Commission that includes representatives from Scotland, Wales and Northern Ireland and in which consumer and public interest nominees are in the majority

- arrangements should be put into place in Scotland, Wales and Northern Ireland to assess policy and legislation emerging from the UK agency and the EC from a territorial perspective and to initiate work on particular territorial issues. The Agency's role should include drafting policy, proposing and drafting legislation, and public education and information within its remit

- the Agency should be responsible for coordinating, monitoring and auditing local food law enforcement activities

- the Agency should coordinate all the research in the food safety, nutrition and consumer protection area

- funding for the Agency should come through the Department of Health budget by a mechanism that is open to public scrutiny.

6.5. The Food Standards Agency

In January 1998 a White paper was published by the government 'The Food Standards Agency: a force for change' which set out detailed proposals for a Food Standards Agency which **'will promote high standards throughout the food chain, from the point of production to the point of consumption. It will be a powerful new body, dealing with a complex area and a wide range of interest groups, from producers, manufacturers and retailers to scientific experts, public health professionals and, most importantly, consumers.'**

At present there is a dissipation regarding the responsibility, enforcement and monitoring of various aspects of food policy. MAFF has the main responsibility for issues concerning food standards, chemical safety of food, labelling, food technology and meat and milk hygiene through a number of executive Agencies including the Meat Hygiene Service and the Milk Hygiene Inspectorate while the Department of Health takes a lead on food hygiene, microbiological safety and nutrition. Local authorities, through Trading Standard Officers and Environmental Health Officers, are responsible for enforcement of the Food Safety Act 1990 and surveillance of the microbiological safety of food is the responsibility of PHLS, CDSCs and health authorities. There has been a need for some years to coordinate and rationalise these functions and responsibilities, preferably in one public body, but it has only been since the recent BSE crisis with its implications both for human health and the economy of the country (especially its farming community) that the driving force has been apparent in government circles.

The guiding principles for the Food Standards Agency are set out in the White paper:

- the essential aim of the Agency is the protection of public health in relation to food

- the Agency's assessments of food standards and safety will be unbiased and based on the best available scientific advice, provided by experts invited in their own right to give independent advice

- the Agency will make decisions and take action on the basis that: the Agency's decisions and actions should be proportionate to the risk; pay due regard to costs as well as to benefits to those affected by them; avoid over-regulation; and that the Agency should act independently of specific sectoral interests

- the Agency will strive to ensure that the public have adequate, clearly presented information to allow them to make informed choices. In doing this, the Agency will aim to avoid raising unjustified alarm

- the Agency's decision making process will be open, transparent and consultative, so that interested parties, including representatives of the public, have opportunity to make their views known; can see the basis on which decisions have been taken; are able to reach an informed judgement about the quality of the Agency's processes and decisions

- before taking action, the Agency will consult widely, including representatives of those who would be affected, unless the need for urgent action to protect public health makes this impossible

- in its decisions and actions, the Agency will aim to achieve clarity and consistency of approach

- the Agency's decisions and actions will take full account of the obligations of the UK under domestic and international law

- the Agency will aim for efficiency and economy in delivering an effective operation.

The White Paper sets out various aspects of food hygiene and food safety that the Food Standards Agency will address. The Agency will:

- integrate the responsibility of both MAFF and DoH in advising Ministers on all aspects of food hygiene and microbiological safety of food policy

- initiate any legislative action required to ensure food hygiene and safety

- coordinate EU and UK food law, as required, taking a proactive role in development of EU policy

- commission and coordinate research and surveillance in microbiological food safety and related areas

- provide ownership of the Meat Hygiene Service, Dairy Hygiene Inspectorate and related bodies in Northern Ireland and their responsibilities

- identify and set standards for the management of local investigations of food-borne outbreaks

- maintain a strategic overview of human and animal surveillance

- coordinate and commission food surveillance programmes

- provide the means of overcoming local boundaries in terms of resources in the case of a widespread outbreak

- take responsibility for the Food Hazard Warning System and liaison with Chief Medical officers, as required

- maintain powers to step in when local management of an outbreak has proven to be ineffective.

This White Paper has been in a consultative phase during 1998 and will probably not become law until 2000 but at the minimum it sets out clear principles by which the increasing numbers of food poisoning cases will be addressed in future.

6.6. EU Food Safety Legislation

Since the introduction of the single European market in 1992, the EU has had a major influence on future food legislation in the UK and other member states. The great majority of secondary legislation concerning food in the UK is initiated by EU negotiations implemented or awaiting implementation throughout the Community. They include Directives concerning the hygiene of premises, processes and personnel involved in the production of specific foods including meat, eggs, milk, fish and their products. There are also directives that deal with related food safety matters such as novel food products and irradiation of foods.

6.7. Conclusion

Over recent years it has become obvious to all those involved in food production, manufacture and public health that the laws regarding food safety and related issues have not been affecting the rise in the reported incidence of food-poisoning in the general population. The Food Act (1990) did address some issues of concern. It is hoped that the introduction of The Food Standards Agency will rationalise the present responsibilities for monitoring and enforcing food legalisation and provide EHOs and others involved in enforcement with new powers which will result in a decrease in reported cases of gastrointestinal disease and provide safer food for the population as a whole.

References and further reading

Advisory Committee on the Microbiological Safety of Food. (1993). *Interim Report on Campylobacter.* HMSO. UK.

Baird-Parker, A.C. (1990). Foodborne salmonellosis. *The Lancet*, Volume 336, pp.1231-1235.

Cliver, D.O. (Ed). (1990). *Foodborne diseases.* Academic Press. San Diego, Calif. USA.

Phillips, C.A. (1996). Review: Modified atmosphere packaging and its effect on the microbiological quality and safety of produce. *International Journal of Food Science and Technology.* Volume 31, pp. 463-479.

Roberts, T.A., Baird-Parker, A.C. and Tompkin, R.B. (Eds). (1996). *Microorganisms in Foods V: Characteristics of Microbial Pathogens.* ICMSF. Blackie Academic and Professional. London: UK.

The Food Standards Agency: a force for change. (1998). The Stationary Office: London.

The Pennington Report. (1997). Report on the circumstances leading to the 1996 outbreak of infection with *E. coli* O157 in Central Scotland, the implications for food safety and the lessons to be learned. The Stationary Office: Edinburgh.

Wall, P.G., de Louvois, J., Gilbert, R.J. and Rowe, B. (1996). Food poisoning: notifications, laboratory reports and outbreaks - what do the statistics mean and where do they come from? *Communicable Disease Review*, Volume 6, Number 7, pp. 93-100.